Low Carb

Top Recipes for Rapid Weight Loss

©Marc Reid

Forward

I would like to thank you for purchasing "Low Carb: 1 Year of Low Carb Recipes for Rapid Weight Loss" and congratulate you for taking the steps to improve your health and wellbeing.

To say that the Low Carb diet is life-changing would be an understatement. Following the Low Carb diet will allow you take control of your health and the benefits that will spill over to all parts of your life. Of course you can expect to see physical changes like definite weight loss and an increase in stamina and strength, and just generally feeling more comfortable in your own skin.

This book will use a step-wise approach to take you through the Low Carb journey and further beyond into the practical application of making healthy and super tasty recipes. The Low Carb diet expounds on a practical and sustainable way to nourish our bodies to maintain lifelong health, physical performance and overall wellness.

As you embark on this health journey, I hope it leads you to a life of pure health bliss and vitality as it has for so many Low Carb devotees.

Table of Contents

Lunch Recipes

Introduction

"Our bodies are our gardens – our wills are our gardeners."

~William Shakespeare

The Low Carb Diets a simple approach to eating whole, unprocessed foods with a focus on nutrient rich vegetables, high-quality, unprocessed meats and heart healthy fats.

Most people on a low-fat diet end up taking in more carbs, especially processed ones, and in turn are hungry all the time. By filling up on whole, low carb foods and ditching the processed grains, sugars, and carbs, you will satiate your appetite while dropping the extra pounds.

This diet will not only change the way you feel about food, it will also change your habits and your cravings. You will experience increased energy levels, improved mental focus and clarity, as well as better sleep.

Sound too good to be true? Give it a try and see for yourself!

Whether you've never heard of the Low Carb diet or you're a veteran who needs some inspiration when it comes to recipes, this book is here to help you to expand your horizons.

The Truth about Carbs

Refined grains and sugars are the biggest sources of carbs and a major cause of inflammation in the American diet, so these are the most important exclusions from the Low Carb Diet plan. High consumption of refined grains (white flour) and sugar is linked with higher risk for myriad diseases, everything from heart disease, stroke, Alzheimer's, and diabetes. Legumes are also high in starch, and they have certain types of fibre that are problematic for some people, so they too are excluded for this portion of the program. Dairy is another common source of dietary sensitivities, in addition to the fact that most milk products in the US today come from grain-fed cows, some of which are treated with hormones. Alcohol is also highly inflammatory, and linked with many serous health conditions.

By following this program for a month, you'll give yourself a chance to see how potentially problematic food groups like dairy, grains, and legumes are affecting your health. Some people can eat moderate amounts of low-fat dairy and whole grains with no problem; others can't, and experience symptoms like bloating, abdominal pain, and fatigue without knowing why. The only way to find out is to try at least a month without these foods and see how you feel. Foods like refined grains and sugar are problematic for *everyone*, because they increase risk factors for chronic illnesses like heart disease, obesity, and diabetes. By cutting these out, you'll likely lose weight and reduce some of the related risk factors. Finally, by eating a lower-carb, higher protein diet, you'll also increase your body's capacity to burn fat as an energy source. Some research has shown that eating a diet lower in carbohydrates and higher in protein than the average American diet aids in weight loss and helps increase the body's ability to utilize fat stores as energy.

There are three other important parts of this program: drink plenty of water (your body needs to be fully hydrated in order to efficiently burn fat), get physical activity (at least 30 minutes to 1 hour every day), and don't step on the scale or take any body measurements. By eliminating grains and sugar, you will automatically eliminate most of the unhealthy foods in your diet, and very likely lose weight. But, sustainable weight loss takes weeks, not days. Your weight can fluctuate as much as 5 pounds in one day, and trying to track your progress with a scale will lead to added stress and take your focus away from the larger goal of better overall health.

Strategies for Success

The goal is not to eat this diet for 30 days and then return to an average American diet full of processed food and soda. The idea is to build new habits that you can sustain for the rest of your life. A great opportunity for this is **finding new snack foods**. Americans tend to snack on a lot of sugary snacks full of refined grains and unhealthy fats. Cookies, candy bars, energy drinks, sodas…all of these provide a quick burst of energy – often leaving with a sugar crash half an hour later – but put you on the fast track to worse health in the future.

Try to find new snack combinations that are tasty, easy to prepare, and convenient to eat on the go. Hard boiled eggs, organic beef jerky, a handful or nuts and dried fruit, an apple with almond butter, raw vegetables dipped in homemade dressing, olives…there are dozens of options to keep you fuelled and on track. Check out the chapter on low carb snacks and make them in advanced so you have a batch for the entire week.

The Low Carb emphasizes protein, but it's important to **choose your proteins thoughtfully**. As much as you can, focus on chicken, turkey, fish, and eggs to supply lean protein in your diet. Make red meat an occasional treat, since current scientific evidence suggests that higher consumption of red meat is linked with a higher risk for heart disease and some cancers. When you do buy beef or lamb, it's very important to get organic, 100% grass-fed meat. Research has shown that the type of fat differs in grass-fed and grain-fed meats, and grass-fed is better for us and the animals.

Decide what you're going to cook a few days in advance, so you can prep ingredients ahead of time and have meals and snacks ready *before* you get super hungry. Slow-cooker stews can be started in the morning and will be ready when you get home from work. Many dishes can be made the day before and reheated. And things like salads are often quick to throw together. Knowing what you have on hand and what you'll make with it will help you stick to your Low Carb Diet.

As part of planning ahead, **take any high carbohydrate foods out of your house**, or at the very least, put them out of sight and each reach. This month will be challenging at times, and you can make it easier on yourself by making it harder to break the rules. You're more likely to eat cookies that you left sitting on your counter than to get dressed, drive to the store, and buy cookies. Our willpower is limited, so remove temptation ahead of time when you can.

It may be challenging, but the Low Carb diet is a great chance to try **new foods and recipes**. Look for recipes from cuisines that don't typically use a lot of grains or legumes, like Thai or Chinese stir-fries and South Asian curries. Take a familiar Low Carb-friendly dish, like beef stew or scrambled eggs, and look for ways to give it a fresh twist with new spices, a different mixture of vegetables, or another culture's take on it.

Finally, **surround yourself with support**. Team up with a friend, spouse, or co-worker who wants to try the Low Carb Diet. You'll be less likely to stop if you're doing it with someone else. Look up the dozens of Low Carb blogs and forums online and join the virtual community. Plan rewards for yourself through the month that don't involve food: a movie, sleeping in, dates with friends, a trip to your favourite store – whatever it is that gives you motivation. Good luck on this valuable step to a healthier you.

Breakfast Recipes

Anaheim pepper Gruyere Waffles

Ingredients

1 small Anaheim pepper

3 eggs

1/4 cup cream cheese

1/4 cup Gruyere cheese

1 Tbsp. coconut flour

1 tsp. Metamucil powder

1 tsp. baking powder

Salt and pepper to taste

Directions

1. In a blender, mix together all ingredients except for the cheese and Anaheim pepper.
2. Once the ingredients are mixed well, add cheese and pepper. Blend well until all ingredients are unit well.
3. Heat your waffle iron; pour on the waffle mix and cook 5-6 minutes.
4. Serve hot.

Servings: 2

Cooking Times

Total Time: 15 minutes

Amount Per Serving

Calories 223, 55

Total Fat 17,25g 27%

Total Carbohydrates 5,53g 2%

Fiber 0,33g 1%

Sugar 1,56g

Protein 11,6g 23%

Anchovy, Spinach and Asparagus Omelet

Ingredients

2 organic eggs

3/4 cup of spinach

2 oz. anchovy in olive oil

4 marinated asparagus

Celtic Sea salt

Freshly ground black pepper

Directions

1. Preheat the oven to 375 F.
2. In the bottom of the baking pan place the anchovy.
3. In a bowl, beat the eggs and pour on top of the fish. Add the spinach and the chopped asparagus on top.
4. Season with salt and pepper to taste.
5. Bake in preheated oven for about 10 minutes.
6. Serve hot.

Servings: 2

Cooking Times

Total Time: 15 minutes

Amount Per Serving

Calories 83, 24

Total Fat 4,91g 8%

Total Carbohydrates 2,28g <1%

Fiber 0,86g 3%

Sugar 0,23g

Protein 7,7g 15%

Autumn Pumpkin Bread

Ingredients

3 egg whites

1/2 cup coconut milk

1 1/2 cup almond flour

1/2 cup pumpkin puree

2 tsp. baking powder

1 1/2 tsp. Pumpkin pie spice

1/2 tsp. Kosher Salt

coconut oil for greasing

Directions

1. Preheat your oven to 350F. Grease a standard bread loaf pan with melted coconut oil.
2. Sift all dry ingredients into a large bowl.
3. In another bowl, add pumpkin puree and coconut milk and mix well. In a separate bowl, beat the egg whites. Fold in egg whites and gently fold into the dough.
4. Spread the dough into the prepared bread pan.
5. Bake the bread for 75 minutes. Once ready, remove bread from the oven and let cool.
6. Slice and serve.

Servings: 8

Cooking Times

Total Time: 1 hour and 25 minutes

Amount Per Serving

Calories 197, 68

Total Fat 16,69g 26%

Total Carbohydrates 8,19g 3%

Fiber 3,31g 13%

Sugar 1,89g

Protein 7,24g 14%

Batter Coated Cheddar Cheese

Ingredients

1 large egg

2 slice Cheddar cheese (3.55 oz.)

1 tsp. ground walnuts

1 tsp. ground flaxseed

2 tsp. almond flour

1 tsp. hemp seeds

1 Tbsp. olive oil

Salt and pepper to taste

Directions

1. In a small bowl, whisk an egg together with the salt and pepper.
2. Heat a tablespoon of olive oil in a frying pan, on medium heat.
3. In a separate bowl, mix the ground flaxseed with the ground walnuts, hemp seeds and the almond flour.
4. Coat the cheddar slices with the egg mix, then roll in the dry mix and fry cheese for about 3 minutes on each side. Serve hot.

Servings: 1

Cooking Times

Total Time: 13 minutes

Amount Per Serving

Calories 509, 86

Total Fat 46,19g 71%

Total Carbohydrates 2,65g <1%

Fiber 0,79g 3%

Protein 21,98g 44%

Chicken Sausage and Pepper Jack Pie

Ingredients

5 egg yolks

1 1/2 chicken sausage

3/4 cup Pepper Jack cheese

1/4 cup coconut flour

2 tsp. lime Juice

1/2 tsp. dried basil

1/4 tsp. baking soda

4 Tbsp. coconut oil

2 Tbsp. coconut water

Kosher salt to taste

Directions

1. Preheat oven to 350F.
2. In a frying pan add the sausages and cook on medium high heat 3-4 minutes. Set aside.
3. Measure out the dry ingredients into a bowl.
4. Separate 5 egg yolks from the whites, then discard of the whites.
5. Beat the egg yolks about 4-5 minutes. Add in coconut oil, coconut water, and lime juice. Continue to beat again until smooth and creamy.
6. Mix the wet ingredients into the dry ingredients slowly. At last, add cheese into the batter.
7. Measure out the batter into 2 ramekins. Poke the sausages into the batter.
8. Bake in preheated oven for 25 minutes. Once ready, serve hot.

Servings: 5

Cooking Times

Total Time: 40 minutes

Amount Per Serving

Calories 294, 15

Total Fat 24,78g 38%

Total Carbohydrates 7,66g 3%

Fiber 0,34g 1%

Protein 11g 22%

Cashew Chocolate & Orange Smoothie

Ingredients

1 cup cashew milk

1 handful of arugula leaves

1 Tbsp. chocolate whey protein powder

1/8 tsp. orange extract

Ice cubes

Directions

1. Place all ingredients in your blender and blend until well united and smooth. Add extra ice and serve.

Servings: 1

Cooking Time: 5 minutes

Amount Per Serving

Calories 44, 97

Total Fat 1,05g 2%

Total Carbohydrates 7,1g 2%

Fiber 2,49g 10%

Sugar 4,4g

Protein 3,97g 8%

Coffee Lowcarbocino

Ingredients

1 cup cold coffee

1/3 cup heavy cream

1/4 tsp. xantham gum

1 tsp. pure vanilla extract

2 Tbsp. Xylitol

6 ice cubes

Directions

1. Place all ingredients in your blender. Blend until all unite well and become smooth. Serve.

Servings: 1

Cooking Times: 5 minutes

Amount Per Serving

Calories 287, 89

Total Fat 29,37g 45%

Total Carbohydrates 2,74g <1%

Fiber 0g 0%

Protein 1,91g 4%

Cheesy Boiled Eggs

Ingredients

3 eggs

2 Tbsp. almond butter, no-stir

2 Tbsp. softened cream cheese

1 tsp. whipping cream

Salt and pepper to taste

Directions

1. In a small saucepan hard boil the eggs.
2. When ready, wash the eggs with cold water, peel and chop them. Place eggs in a bowl; add in the butter, cream cheese and whipping cream.
3. Mix well and add salt and pepper to taste. Serve.

Servings: 2

Cooking Time: 20 minutes

Amount Per Serving

Calories 212, 41

Total Fat 19,88g 31%

Total Carbohydrates 0,75g <1%

Fiber 0g 0%

Protein 7,74g 15%

Mahón Kale Sausage Omelet Pie

Ingredients

10 eggs

1 1/2 cup Mahón cheese (or Cheddar)

3 chicken sausages

3 cups raw chopped Kale leaves

2 1/2 cup mushrooms, chopped

1 Tbsp. garlic powder

2 tsp. hot sauce

1/2 tsp. black pepper and celery seed

salt and pepper to taste

Directions

1. Preheat oven to 400F.
2. Chop up your sausage and mushroom thin and place them in a cast iron skillet. Cook on a medium-high heat for 2-3 minutes.
3. While the sausages are cooking, chop your spinach up. Add in a skillet the mushrooms and spinach.
4. In a meanwhile, in a bowl mix eggs with black pepper and celery seed, hot sauce, and spices. Scramble them well.
5. Mix your sausages, spinach, and mushrooms so that the spinach can wilt fully. Add salt and pepper to taste.
6. Finally, add the cheese to the top.
7. Pour your eggs over the mixture and mix everything well.
8. Stir the mixture for a few seconds, and then put your cast iron skillet in the oven. Bake for 10-12 minutes, and then broil the top for 3-4 minutes.
9. Let cool for a while, cut into 8 slices and serve hot.

Servings: 8

Cooking Times

Total Time: 25 minutes

Amount Per Serving

Calories 266, 11

Total Fat 17,76g 27%

Total Carbohydrates 7,67g 3%

Fiber 0,92g 4%

Protein 19,37g 39%

Monterey Bacon-Scallions Omelet

Ingredients

2 eggs

2 slices cooked bacon

1/4 cup scallions, chopped

1/4 cup Monterey jack cheese

salt and pepper to taste

1 tsp. lard

Directions

1. In a frying pan heat lard in on medium-low heat. Add the eggs, scallions and salt and pepper to taste.
2. Cook for 1-2 minutes; add the bacon and sauté 30 - 45 seconds longer. Turn the heat off on the stove.
3. On top of the bacon place a cheese. Then, take two edges of the omelet and fold them onto the cheese. Hold the edges there for a moment as the cheese has to partially melt. Make the same with the other egg and let cook in a warm pan for a while.
4. Serve hot.

Servings: 2

Cooking Times

Total Time: 15 minutes

Amount Per Serving

Calories 321, 48

Total Fat 28,31g 44%

Total Carbohydrates 1,62g <1%

Fiber 0,33g 1%

Protein 14,37g 29%

Smoked Turkey Bacon and Avocado Muffins

Ingredients

5 eggs

6 slices smoked turkey bacon

1/2 cup almond flour

2 medium Avocados

1/2 cup Cheddar cheese

1 1/2 cup coconut milk

3 spring onions

1 tsp. minced garlic

2 tsp. dried parsley

1/4 tsp. red chili powder

1 1/2 Tbsp. lemon juice

1/4 cup flaxseed

1 1/2 Tbsp. Metamucil powder

1 tsp. baking powder

2 Tbsp. butter

salt and pepper to taste

Directions

1. Preheat oven to 350F.
2. In a frying pan over medium-low heat, cook the bacon with the butter until crisp. Add the spring onions, cheese, and baking powder.
3. In a bowl, mix together coconut milk, eggs, Metamucil powder, almond flour, flax, spices and lemon juice. Switch off the heat and let cool. Then, crumble the bacon and add all of the fat to the egg mixture.
4. Clean and chop avocado and fold into the mixture.
5. Measure out batter into a cupcake tray that's been sprayed or greased with nonstick spray and bake for 25-26 minutes.
6. Once ready, let cool and serve hot or cold.

Servings: 16

Cooking Times

Total Time: 40 minutes

Amount Per Serving

Calories 184, 26

Total Fat 16,4g 25%

Total Carbohydrates 5,51g 2%

Fiber 2,7g 11%

Protein 5,89g 12%

Sour Cream Cheese Pancakes

Ingredients

2 eggs

1/4 cup cream cheese

1 Tbsp. coconut flour

1 tsp. ground ginger

1/2 cup liquid Stevia

coconut oil

sugar-free maple syrup

Directions

1. In a deep bowl, beat together all of the ingredients until smooth.

2. Heat up a frying skillet with oil on medium-high. Ladle the batter and pour in hot oil.

3. Cook on one side and then flip. Top with a sugar-free maple syrup and serve.

Servings: 2

Cooking Times

Total Time: 15 minutes

Amount Per Serving

Calories 170, 78

Total Fat 13,71g 21%

Total Carbohydrates 4,39g 1%

Fiber 0,14g <1%

Protein 6,9g 14%

Spicy Cauliflower with Sujuk Sausages

Ingredients

4 cups frozen cauliflower

8 oz. sujuk sausages sliced (or red pastrami)

1 green pepper, chopped

1 tsp. Cajun seasoning

1/2 onion, chopped

2 Tbsp. minced garlic

2 Tbsp. olive oil

Directions

1. In a frying pan, sauté onion with olive oil for 2-3 minutes.
2. Squeeze the liquid from chopped cauliflower and add it to the pan. Sauté the cauliflower with onion 5-10 minutes.
3. Add in Cajun seasoning and mix. Add in chopped sujuk sausages or pastrami and green peppers.
4. Toss and cook until about 5 minutes. Transfer to the plates. Serve.

Servings: 4

Cooking Times

Total Time: 20 minutes

Amount Per Serving

Calories 181, 57

Total Fat 10,21g

Total Carbohydrates 9,52g

Fiber 2,77g

Protein 14,12g

Strawberry Marjoram Smoothie

Ingredients

1/4 cup fresh or frozen strawberries

2 fresh marjoram leaves

2 Tbsp. heavy cream

1 cup unsweetened coconut milk

1 Tbsp. sugar-free vanilla syrup

1/2 tsp. pure vanilla extract

ice cubes (optional)

Directions

1. Place all ingredients in your blender and mix until become smooth.
2. If you wish you can add the ice cubes. Serve.

Servings: 1

Cooking Time: 5 minutes

Amount Per Serving

Calories 292, 35

Total Fat 29,75g

Total Carbohydrates 6,78g

Protein 2,84g

Vesuvius Scrambled Eggs with Provolone

Ingredients

2 large eggs

3/4 cup Provolone cheese

1.76 oz. air-dried salami

1 tsp. fresh rosemary (chopped)

1 Tbsp. Olive oil

Salt and pepper to taste

Directions

1. In a small pan with olive oil fry the chopped salami.
2. In the meantime, in a small bowl whisk the eggs, then add the salt, pepper and fresh rosemary.
3. Add in the provolone cheese and mix well with a fork.
4. Pour the egg mixture to the pan with salami and cook for about 5 minutes. Serve hot.

Servings: 2

Cooking Time: 10 minutes

Amount Per Serving

Calories 374, 48

Total Fat 30,32g

Total Carbs 2,43g

Fiber 0,27g

Protein 22,45g

Pizza Waffles

Ingredients

Parmesan cheese (4 tablespoons)

Psyllium husk powder (1 tablespoon)

Baking powder (1 teaspoon)

Salt

Cheddar cheese (3 oz.)

Eggs (4, large)

Almond flour (3 tablespoons)

Butter (1 tablespoon, organic)

Italian seasoning (1 teaspoon)-you may use a teaspoon of your preferred spices

Tomato sauce (1/2 cup)

Directions

1. Add all ingredients to a bowl except cheese and tomato sauce. Use mixer or immersion blender to combine until mixture is thick.

2. Heat waffle iron and use mixture to make two waffles.

3. Place waffles onto a lined baking sheet and top with tomato sauce and cheese (divide evenly). Broil for 3 minutes or until cheese melts.

4. Serve.

Servings: 2

Nutritional Information

Calories 525.5

Net Carbs 5g

Fats 41.5g

Protein 29g

Fiber 5.5g

Pancakes and Syrup

Ingredients

For pancakes:

Eggs (4, large)

Erythritol (2 tablespoons)

Baking soda (1/2 teaspoon)

Nut butter of your choice (3/4 cup)

Coconut milk (1/3 cup)

Ghee (2 tablespoons)

Cinnamon powder (1 teaspoon)

For Syrup:

Maple extract (2 tablespoons, sugar-free)

Sukrin Fiber Syrup (1/2 cup)

Directions

1. Add ingredients for syrup to a jar and use spoon to stir until combined thoroughly. Cover jar and put aside until needed.

2. Put eggs, erythritol, baking soda, nut butter, coconut milk and cinnamon powder in a food processor and pulse until blended.

3. Heat ghee in a non-stick skillet and add batter to pot, use about ¼ cup per pancake. Cook until pancake sets then flip and finish cooking; place on a plate.

4. Repeat with remaining batter and plate.

5. Top with syrup and serve.

Servings: 5

Nutritional Information

Calories 401

Net Carbs 3.6g

Fats 32.5g

Protein 12.8g

Fiber 5.3g

Cheesy Bacon and Chive Omelet

Ingredients

Bacon fat (1 teaspoon)

Cheddar cheese (1 oz.)

Salt

Bacon (2 slices, cooked)

Eggs (2, large)

Black pepper

Chives (2 stalks)

Directions

1. Beat eggs together and add pepper and salt to taste. Chop chives and shred cheese.

2. Heat skillet and cook bacon fat until hot.

3. Add eggs to pot and top with chives. Cook until edges start to set then add bacon and cook for 30-60 seconds.

4. Add cheese and use spatula to fold in half. Press to seal and flip over.

5. Warm and serve immediately.

Servings: 1

Nutritional Information

Calories 463

Net Carbs 1g

Fats 39g

Protein 24g

Fiber 0g

Breakfast Quiche

Ingredients

Coconut oil (3 tablespoons)

5 whole eggs

8 slices of bacon, cooked and chopped

100ml cream

Baby spinach, roughly chopped (2 cups)

Red pepper, chopped (1 cup)

Green pepper, chopped (1 cup)

Yellow onion, chopped (1 cup)

2 cloves of garlic, minced

Mushrooms, chopped (1 cup)

100g cheddar cheese, grated

salt to taste

Directions

1. Preheat oven at 375F

2. In a large bowl, mix all vegetables including the mushrooms together.

3. In another small bowl, whisk the 5 eggs with the cream

4. Carefully scoop the veggie mixture into a muffin pan coated with cooking spray, top with egg and cheese filling up to ¾ of the muffin tins. Sprinkle with chopped bacon on top.

5. Place in the oven to bake for 15 minutes or until the top of the quiche are firm.

6. Let it cook for a few minutes before serving.

Servings: 5

Nutritional Information (1 small quiche)

Calories: 210

Net Carbs: 5g

Fat: 13g

Protein: 6g

Bacon Avocado Breakfast Muffins

Ingredients

Bacon (5 slices)

Almond flour (1/2 cup)

Psyllium husk powder (1 ½ tablespoons)

Colby Jack cheese (4.5 oz.)

Garlic (1 teaspoon, diced)

Chives (1 teaspoon, dried)

Salt

Lemon juice (1 ½ tablespoons)

Eggs (5)

Butter (2 tablespoons, organic)

Flaxseed meal (1/4 cup)

Avocados (2, cubed)

Spring onions (3)

Cilantro (1 teaspoon, dried)

Red chili flakes (1/4 teaspoon)

Coconut milk (1 ½ cup, from box)

Black Pepper

Baking powder (1 teaspoon)

Directions

1. Add flour, spices, lemon juice, eggs, flaxseed meal and coconut milk to a bowl. Mix together until thoroughly combined.

2. Heat a skillet and cook bacon until crispy then add the butter and avocado.

3. Add mixture to batter in bowl and mix together.

4. Set oven to 350 F and grease cupcake molds.

5. Add batter to molds and bake for 26 minutes. Take from oven and cool before removing from mold.

6. Serve. Store leftovers in fridge.

Servings: 16

Nutritional Information

Calories 163

Net Carbs 1.5g

Fats 14.1g

Protein 6.1g

Fiber 3.3g

Chicharrones con Huevos (Pork Rind & Eggs)

Ingredients

Bacon (4 slices)

Pork Rinds (1.5 oz.)

Avocado (1, cubed)

Onion (1/4, chopped)

Salt

Eggs (5)

Tomato (1, chopped)

Jalapeno pepper (2, seeds removed and chopped)

Cilantro (1/4 cup, chopped)

Black pepper

Directions

1. Heat skillet and cook bacon until slightly crisp. Remove from pot and put aside on paper towels.

2. Add pork rinds to pot along with onion, tomatoes, pepper and cook for 3 minutes until onions are soft and clear.

3. Add cilantro, stir together gently and add eggs. Scramble eggs and then add avocado and fold.

4. Serve.

Servings: 3

Nutritional Information

Calories 508

Net Carbs 5g

Fats 43g

Protein 24.7g

Fiber 5.3g

Red Pepper, Mozzarella and Bacon Frittata

Ingredients

Olive oil (1 tablespoon)

Parsley (2 tablespoons, chopped)

Mozzarella cheese (4 oz., cubed)

Bell pepper (1, red, chopped)

Heavy cream (1/4 cup)

Salt

Bacon (7 slices)

Bella mushrooms (4 caps, large)

Basil (1/2 cup, chopped)

Goat cheese (2 oz., grated)

Eggs (9)

Parmesan cheese (1/4 cup, grated)

Black pepper

Directions

1. Set oven to 350 °F.

2. Chop red pepper, bacon, basil and mushroom. Slice mozzarella into cubes and put aside.

3. Heat olive oil in a skillet until it slightly smokes then add bacon and cook for 5 minutes until browned.

4. Add red pepper and cook for 2 minutes until soft. While pepper cooks, add cream, parmesan cheese, eggs and black pepper to a bowl and whisk to combine.

5. Add mushrooms to pot, stir and cook for 5 minutes until soaked in fat. Add basil, cook for 1 minute then add mozzarella.

6. Put in egg mixture and use spoon to move ingredients around so that the egg gets on the bottom of pan.

7. Top with goat cheese and place in oven for 8 minutes then broil for 6 minutes.

8. Use knife to pry frittata edges from pan and place on a plate and slice.

9. Serve.

Servings: 6

Nutritional Information

Calories 408

Net Carbs 2.4g

Fats 31.2g

Protein 19.2g

Fiber 0.8g

Cheese and Sausage Pies

Ingredients

Cheddar cheese (3/4 cup, grated)

Coconut oil (1/4 cup)

Egg yolks (5)

Rosemary (1/2 teaspoon)

Baking soda (1/4 teaspoon)

Chicken sausage (1 ½)

Coconut flour (1/4 cup)

Coconut milk (2 tablespoons)

Lemon juice (2 teaspoons)

Cayenne pepper (1/4 teaspoon)

Kosher salt (1/8 teaspoon)

Directions

1. Set oven to 350 F.

2. Chop sausage, heat skillet and cook sausage. While sausages cook combine all dry ingredients in a bowl. In another bowl combine lemon juice, oil and coconut milk. Add liquids to dry mixture and add ½ cup of cheese; fold to combine and put into 2 ramekins.

3. Add cooked sausages to batter and use spoon to push into mixture.

4. Bake for 25 minutes until golden on top. Top with leftover cheese and broil for 4 minutes.

5. Serve warm.

Servings: 2

Nutritional Information

Calories 711

Net Carbs 5.8g

Fats 65.3g

Protein 34.3g

Fiber 11.5g

Vanilla Chia Oatmeal

Ingredients

Chia seeds (1/4 cup)

Coconut flakes (1/3 cup, unsweetened)

Vanilla (1 teaspoon, sugar free)

Almond milk (1 cup, unsweetened)

Stevia extract (10 drops)

Coconut (1/4 cup, shredded, unsweetened)

Almonds (1/3 cup, flaked)

Heavy whipping cream (1/2 cup)

Erythritol (2 tablespoons)

Directions

1. Place almond and coconut flakes in a pot and toast for 3 minutes until fragrant.

2. Place toasted ingredients into a bowl along with chia seeds, erythritol and shredded coconut; mix together to combine.

3. Top with milk and stir. You can use hot or cold milk based on your preference.

4. Add vanilla and stevia, stir and set aside for 5-10 minutes.

5. Serve. May be topped with fresh berries.

Servings: 2

Nutritional Information

Calories 359

Net Carbs 5g

Fats 30.4g

Protein 9.4 g

Fiber 10.5g

Breakfast Berry Shake

Ingredients

Mixed berries (3/4 cup)

Almond milk (1 cup)

All-natural peanut butter (1 tablespoon)

Protein powder (1 tablespoon)

Cinnamon powder (1/4 teaspoons)

Ginger, minced (1/4 teaspoons)

Directions

1. Place all the ingredients in a blender and mix until smooth.

Servings: 3

Nutritional Information

Calories: 319

Net Carbs: 9g

Fat: 15g

Protein: 28g

Breakfast Tacos

Ingredients

Eggs (6)

Bacon (3 strips)

Cheddar cheese (1 oz., shredded)

Mozzarella cheese (1 cup, shredded)

Butter (2 tablespoons)

Avocado (1/2, cubed)

Salt

Black pepper

Directions

1. Cook bacon until crisp, put aside until needed.

2. Heat a non-stick pan and place 1/3 cup mozzarella into pan and cook for 3 minutes until browned around the edges. Place a wooden spoon across a bowl or pot and use tongs to lift cheese 'taco from pot. Repeat with leftover cheese.

3. Melt butter in a skillet and scramble eggs; use pepper and salt to season.

4. Spoon eggs into hardened shells and top with avocado and bacon.

5. Top with cheddar and serve.

Servings: 2

Nutritional Information

Calories 443

Net Carbs 3g

Fats 36.2g

Protein 25.7 g

Fiber 1.7g

Raspberry & Cacao Breakfast Pudding

Ingredients

Cacao powder (1 tablespoon)

Raspberry (1/4 cups)

Chia seeds (3 tablespoon)

Almond milk (1 cup)

Agave or Xylitol (1 teaspoon)

Directions

1. In a small bowl, combine the almond milk and cacao powder. Stir well.

2. Add the chia seeds to the bowl and let it rest for 5 minutes.

3. Using a fork, fluff the chia and cacao mixture and then place in the fridge to chill for at least 30 minutes.

4. Serve with raspberries and a drizzle of agave on top

Servings: 1

Nutritional Information

Calories 230

Net Carbs 4g

Fats 20g

Protein 15 g

Orange Cinnamon Scones

Ingredients

For Scones:

Heavy cream (1/3 cup)

Butter (1/4 cup, unsalted, cubed)

Coconut oil (2 tablespoons)

Golden Flaxseed (1 tablespoon)

Cinnamon (1 ½ teaspoons)

Xanthan (1/4 teaspoon)

Salt (1/4 teaspoon)

Coconut flour (8 tablespoons)

Erythitol (1/4 cup)

Eggs (2)

Maple syrup (2 tablespoons)-recipe above

Baking powder (1 ½ teaspoons)

Vanilla (1 teaspoon)

Stevia (1/4 teaspoon)

Orange zest (from 1 orange)

For Icing:

Stevia (20 drops)

Orange juice (1 tablespoon)

Coconut butter (1/4 cup)

Directions

1. Set oven to 400 F.

2. Place all dry ingredients in a bowl except xanthan and 1 tablespoon flour. Add butter and oil to dry mix and stir to combine.

3. Combine sweetener and eggs until thoroughly mixed and light in color. Put in maple syrup, remaining flour, xanthan gum, heavy cream and vanilla; mix until combined and thick.

4. Add wet mixture to dry, reserving 2 tablespoons of liquids, mix together and add cinnamon and use hands to form mixture into dough. Shape into a ball and press into a cake like shape. Slice into 8 pieces.

5. Place onto a lined baking sheet and use reserved liquid to brush the top of scones.

6. Bake for 15 minutes, remove from oven and cool.

7. Prepare icing and drizzle over scones before serving.

Servings: 8

Nutritional Information

Calories 232

Net Carbs 3.3g

Fats 20g

Protein 3.3 g

Fiber 4.3g

Buttermilk Seed Rusks

Ingredients

½ cup butter, melted

1 cup buttermilk

4 eggs

1 cup almond flour

1 cup ground flax

2 cups desiccated coconut

1 cup mixed seeds

2 ½ tsp. baking powder

1 tsp. salt

½ cup Xylitol

Directions

1. Preheat oven at 350F
2. In a bowl, combine the yogurt, butter, and eggs.
3. Slowly add the dry ingredients and stir well to make a batter.
4. Carefully transfer the mixture into a baking tray and cook in the oven for 45 minutes.
5. Allow to cool down before slicing it into 30 rusk shapes.
6. Place on a wire rack upside down, and cook in the oven again for 90 minutes at 210F.

Servings: 30

Nutritional Info (1 rusk)

Calories: 119

Net Carbs: 17g

Fat: 3g

Protein: 2g

Caprese Stack

Ingredients

3 slices mozzarella cheese

2 large slices of tomato

4 fresh basil leaves

salt and pepper

1 tsp. olive oil

Directions

1. On a plate, stack the mozzarella cheese, tomato, and basil.
2. Season with salt and pepper and drizzle with olive oil

Nutritional Info (per stack)

Calories: 186

Net Carbs: 5g

Fat: 10g

Protein: 6g

Easy Pancakes

Ingredients

1 tbsp. melted butter

2 eggs

5 tbsp. full-fat milk

1 tbsp. xylitol

½ tsp. salt

2 tbsp. coconut flour

1 tbsp. almond flour

½ tsp. baking powder

Directions

1. In a bowl, whisk the eggs with the milk, salt, xylitol, and melted butter (room temp.)
2. Add the coconut and almond flour to the mixture, along with the baking powder. Mix well.
3. Heat a non-stick pan over medium fire and scoop 3 tbsp. of the batter to make pancakes.
4. Flip the pancake when bubbles start to form and cook until golden brown.
5. Serve with ½ cup of berries on the side.

Servings: 2

Nutritional Info (1 pc.)

Calories: 194

Net Carbs: 30g

Fat: 13g

Protein: 31g

Mug Bread

Ingredients

1 tbsp. coconut flour

3 tbsp. almond flour

1 tsp. baking powder

1 whole egg

1 tsp. melted butter

3 tbsp. water

a pinch of salt

Directions

1. Add all the dry ingredients in a bowl then add the egg and water and mix well make sure there are no lumps in your mixture.
2. Pour the melted butter in the cup you are going to use. You can also use the cup to melt the butter to begin with, but make sure not to over heat the butter; 5 seconds in the microwave should be more than enough. Now swirl the butter around the cup make sure to coat the inside of the cup then pour the butter into the bread mix and combine.
3. Pour the mix in your cup and microwave for 1.5 minutes. if you are planning on doubling the mix I would suggest using a bigger wider mug or the mix will not cook all the way through. Don't microwave for more than 3 min or the mix will end up hard.
4. Once you have removed it from the mug, you can then slice it into rounds and place it in the toaster to crisp it up a little.

Servings: 1

Nutritional Info (1 serving)

Calories: 238

Net Carbs: 2.6g

Fat: 19g

Protein: 13g

Veggie Scramble

Ingredients

4 egg whites

1 egg yolk

2 tbsp. almond milk

1 cup spinach

1 tomato, chopped

½ white onion, chopped

3 fresh basil leaves, chopped

salt and pepper to taste

ghee

Directions

1. In a bowl, whisk the egg yolk and whites with the milk. Stir well.
2. Heat the ghee on a pan over medium heat. Add the onions and sauté until fragrant.
3. Throw in the tomato to the pan with the spinach and cook until the spinach is almost wilted.
4. Pour the egg mixture to the spinach and cook until firm or until the egg sets. Stir constantly.
5. Season with salt and pepper.
6. Serve warm

Nutritional Info (per serving)

Calories: 203

Net Carbs: 18g

Fat: 5g

Protein: 20g

Egg Pesto Scramble

Ingredients

3 eggs

1 tbsp. pesto sauce

1 tbsp. olive oil

2 tbsp. sour cream

Directions

1. Whisk the eggs in a bowl and season with salt and pepper.
2. Heat a non-stick pan over low heat. Drizzle with olive oil and pour the eggs. Constantly whisk the eggs while cooking.
3. Add the pesto mixture to the eggs and stir well.
4. Turn off the fire and mix in the sour cream. Combine well.
5. Serve with 1/2 cup mashed avocado.

Servings: 1

Nutritional Info (per serving)

Calories: 467

Net Carbs: 3.3g

Fat: 41.5g

Protein: 20.4g

Cheesy Low Carb Bread

Ingredients

125g full-fat cream cheese

1 cup cheddar cheese, grated

3 large eggs

1 tsp. apple cider vinegar

2 cups almond flour

2 tsp. baking powder

1 tsp. mustard powder

1 tsp. salt

Directions

1. Preheat oven at 375F
2. Combine all the ingredients in a bowl with a hand mixer, except the cheddar cheese.
3. Add the cheddar cheese to the mixture and combine using a spatula or a fork. Be careful not to mush the cheese.
4. Line a bread tin with well-greased baking paper and bake in the oven for 45 minutes.

Nutritional Info (per serving)

Calories: 495

Net Carbs: 6.5g

Fat: 9.6g

Protein: 19.7g

Lemon Cheesecake Breakfast Mousse

Ingredients

3 tbsp. cream cheese

1 tbsp. lemon juice

50ml heavy cream (look for those with zero carbs)

100ml Yoghurt

1tbsp. Xylitol

1/8 tsp. salt

2 tbsp. whey protein

Directions

1. Blend cream cheese and lemon juice in a bowl until smooth.
2. Add heavy cream and blend until whipped. Gently add in yoghurt.
3. Taste and adjust sweetener if needed.
4. Serve with ¼ cup berry coulis.

Berry Breakfast Shake

Ingredients

¾ cup mixed berries

1 cup almond milk

1 tbsp. all-natural peanut butter

1 tbsp. protein powder

¼ tsp. cinnamon powder

¼ tsp. ginger, minced

Directions

1.   Place all the ingredients in a blender and mix until smooth.

Servings: 1

Nutritional Info (per serving)

Calories: 319

Net Carbs: 9g

Fat: 15g

Protein: 28g

Cacao and Raspberry Pudding

Ingredients

1 tbsp. cacao powder

¼ cup raspberry

3 tbsp. chia seeds

1 cup almond milk

1 tsp. agave

Directions

2. In a small bowl, combine the almond milk and cacao powder. Stir well.
3. Add the chia seeds to the bowl and let it rest for 5 minutes.
4. Using a fork, fluff the chia and cacao mixture and then place in the fridge to chill for at least 30 minutes.
5. Serve with raspberries and a drizzle of agave on top

Coco and Blueberry Smoothie

Ingredients

½ cup blueberries

½ cup coconut cream

1 tbsp. coconut oil

½ cup almond milk, vanilla flavor

3 ice cubes

Directions

1. Place all the ingredients in a blender and mix until you achieve a smooth consistency.

Servings: 2

Nutrition info for one serving:

Calories, 295

Grams of fat, 24

Grams of protein, 13

Grams carbs, 6

Grams fibre 1

Creamy Chocolate Milk

Ingredients

16 ounces unsweetened almond milk

1 teaspoon xylitol

4 ounces heavy cream

1 scoop Whey Chocolate Isolate powder

1/2 cup crushed ice (optional: add if you like a thick drink, but the flavour will be less intense.)

Directions

1. Put all ingredients in blender and blend until smooth.

Servings: 2

Nutrition info for one serving:

292 calories,

25 grams of fat,

15 grams of protein,

4 carbs.

Blueberry Almond Smoothie

Ingredients

16 ounces unsweetened almond milk

1 teaspoon xylitol

4 ounces heavy cream

1/4 cup frozen unsweetened blueberries

1 scoop Whey Vanilla protein powder

Directions

1. Put all ingredients in blender and blend until smooth.
2. Add a little water if it becomes too thick.
3. Measure those blueberries as they add more carbs.

Servings: 2

Nutrition info for one serving:

302 calories,

25 grams of fat,

15 grams of protein,

6 grams carbs,

1 grams fibre.

Mozzarella, Red Pepper & Bacon Frittata

Ingredients

Olive oil (1 tablespoon)

Parsley (2 tablespoons, chopped)

Mozzarella cheese (4 oz., cubed)

Bell pepper (1, red, chopped)

Heavy cream (1/4 cup)

Salt

Bacon (7 slices)

Bella mushrooms (4 caps, large)

Basil (1/2 cup, chopped)

Goat cheese (2 oz., grated)

Eggs (9)

Parmesan cheese (1/4 cup, grated)

Black pepper

Directions

1. Set oven to 350°F.
2. Chop red pepper, bacon, basil and mushroom. Slice mozzarella into cubes and put aside.
3. Heat olive oil in a skillet until it slightly smokes then add bacon and cook for 5 minutes until browned.
4. Add red pepper and cook for 2 minutes until soft. While pepper cooks, add cream, parmesan cheese, eggs and black pepper to a bowl and whisk to combine.

5. Add mushrooms to pot, stir and cook for 5 minutes until soaked in fat. Add basil, cook for 1 minute then add mozzarella.
6. Put in egg mixture and use spoon to move ingredients around so that the egg gets on the bottom of pan.
7. Top with goat cheese and place in oven for 8 minutes then broil for 6 minutes.
8. Use knife to pry frittata edges from pan and place on a plate and slice.
9. Serve.

Servings: 6

Nutritional Information

Calories 408

Net Carbs 2.4g

Fats 31.2g

Protein 19.2g

Fiber 0.8g

Rosemary, Sausage & Cheese Pies

Ingredients

Cheddar cheese (3/4 cup, grated)

Coconut oil (1/4 cup)

Egg yolks (5)

Rosemary (1/2 teaspoon)

Baking soda (1/4 teaspoon)

Chicken sausage (1 ½)

Coconut flour (1/4 cup)

Coconut milk (2 tablespoons)

Lemon juice (2 teaspoons)

Cayenne pepper (1/4 teaspoon)

Kosher salt (1/8 teaspoon)

Directions

1. Set oven to 350 ̊F.
2. Chop sausage, heat skillet and cook sausage. While sausages cook combine all dry ingredients in a bowl. In another bowl combine lemon juice, oil and coconut milk. Add liquids to dry mixture and add ½ cup of cheese; fold to combine and put into 2 ramekins.
3. Add cooked sausages to batter and use spoon to push into mixture.
4. Bake for 25 minutes until golden on top. Top with leftover cheese and broil for 4 minutes.
5. Serve warm.

Servings: 2

Nutritional Information

Calories 711

Net Carbs 5.8g

Fats 65.3g

Protein 34.3g

Fiber 11.5g

Kale Sausage Omelet Pie

Ingredients

10 eggs

1 1/2 cup Mahón cheese (or Cheddar)

3 chicken sausages

3 cups raw chopped Kale leaves

2 1/2 cup mushrooms, chopped

1 Tbsp. garlic powder

2 tsp. hot sauce

1/2 tsp. black pepper and celery seed

salt and pepper to taste

Directions

1. Preheat oven to 400F.
2. Chop up your sausage and mushroom thin and place them in a cast iron skillet. Cook on a medium-high heat for 2-3 minutes.
3. While the sausages are cooking, chop your spinach up. Add in a skillet the mushrooms and spinach.
4. In a meanwhile, in a bowl mix eggs with black pepper and celery seed, hot sauce, and spices. Scramble them well.
5. Mix your sausages, spinach, and mushrooms so that the spinach can wilt fully. Add salt and pepper to taste.
6. Finally, add the cheese to the top.
7. Pour your eggs over the mixture and mix everything well.
8. Stir the mixture for a few seconds, and then put your cast iron skillet in the oven. Bake for 10-12 minutes, and then broil the top for 3-4 minutes.
9. Let cool for a while, cut into 8 slices and serve hot.

Servings: 8

Cooking Time: 25 minutes

Amount Per Serving

Calories 266, 11

Total Fat 17,76g

Total Carbohydrates 7,67g

Fiber 0,92g

Protein 19,37g

Bacon, Scallions & Monterey Omelet

Ingredients

2 eggs

2 slices cooked bacon

1/4 cup scallions, chopped

1/4 cup Monterey jack cheese

salt and pepper to taste

1 tsp. lard

Directions

1. In a frying pan heat lard in on medium-low heat. Add the eggs, scallions and salt and pepper to taste.
2. Cook for 1-2 minutes; add the bacon and sauté 30 - 45 seconds longer. Turn the heat off on the stove.
3. On top of the bacon place a cheese. Then, take two edges of the omelet and fold them onto the cheese. Hold the edges there for a moment as the cheese has to partially melt. Make the same with the other egg and let cook in a warm pan for a while.
4. Serve hot.

Servings: 2

Cooking Time: 15 minutes

Amount Per Serving

Calories 321, 48

Total Fat 28,31g

Total Carbs 1,62g

Fiber 0,33g

Sugar 0,55g

Protein 14,37g

Bacon, Avocado & Smoked Turkey Muffins

Ingredients

5 eggs

6 slices smoked turkey bacon

1/2 cup almond flour

2 medium Avocados

1/2 cup Cheddar cheese

1 1/2 cup coconut milk

3 spring onions

1 tsp. minced garlic

2 tsp. dried parsley

1/4 tsp. red chili powder

1 1/2 Tbsp. lemon juice

1/4 cup flaxseed

1 1/2 Tbsp. Metamucil powder

1 tsp. baking powder

2 Tbsp. butter

salt and pepper to taste

Directions

1. Preheat oven to 350F.
2. In a frying pan over medium-low heat, cook the bacon with the butter until crisp. Add the spring onions, cheese, and baking powder.

3. In a bowl, mix together coconut milk, eggs, Metamucil powder, almond flour, flax, spices and lemon juice. Switch off the heat and let cool. Then, crumble the bacon and add all of the fat to the egg mixture.
4. Clean and chop avocado and fold into the mixture.
5. Measure out batter into a cupcake tray that's been sprayed or greased with nonstick spray and bake for 25-26 minutes.
6. Once ready, let cool and serve hot or cold.

Servings: 16

Cooking Time: 40 minutes

Amount Per Serving

Calories 184

Total Fat 16,4g

Total Carbs 5,51g

Fiber 2,7g

Sugar 0,54g

Protein 5,89g

Cream Cheese Pancakes

Ingredients

2 eggs

1/4 cup cream cheese

1 Tbsp. coconut flour

1 tsp. ground ginger

1/2 cup liquid Stevia

coconut oil

sugar-free maple syrup

Directions

1. In a deep bowl, beat together all of the ingredients until smooth.
2. Heat up a frying skillet with oil on medium-high. Ladle the batter and pour in hot oil.
3. Cook on one side and then flip. Top with a sugar-free maple syrup and serve.

Servings: 16

Cooking Time: 15 minutes

Amount Per Serving

Calories 170, 78

Total Fat 13,71g

Total Carbohydrates 4,39g

Fiber 0,14g

Protein 6,9g

Adorable Pumpkin Flaxseed Muffins

Ingredients

1 egg

1 1/4 cup flaxseeds (ground)

1 cup pumpkin puree

1 Tbs pumpkin pie spice

2 Tbs coconut oil

1/2 cup sweetener of your choice

1 tsp baking powder

2 tsp cinnamon

1/2 tsp apple cider vinegar

1/2 tsp vanilla extract

salt to taste

Directions

1. Preheat your oven to 360°F.
2. First, grind the flaxseeds for several seconds.
3. Put together all the dry ingredients and stir.
4. Then, add your pumpkin puree and mix to combine.
5. Add the vanilla extract and the pumpkin spice.
6. Add in coconut oil, egg and apple vinegar. Add sweetener of your choice and stir again.
7. Add a heaping tablespoon of batter to each lined muffin or cupcake and top with some pumpkin seeds.
8. Bake for about 18 - 20 minutes. Serve hot.

Servings: 10

Cooking Times

Total Time: 20 minutes

Nutrition Facts (per serving)

Total Carbohydrates: 3g

Dietary Fiber: 1g

Net Carbs: 0.9g

Protein: 1g

Total Fat: 5.34g

Calories: 43

Baked Ham and Kale Scrambled Eggs

Ingredients

5 ounces ham diced

2 medium eggs

1 green onion, finely chopped

1/2 cups kale leaves, chopped

1 garlic clove, crushed

1 green chilli, finely chopped

4 ready-roasted peppers

pinch cayenne pepper

1 Tbsp olive oil

1/2 can water

Directions

1. Heat oven to 360F.
2. Heat the oil in a small ovenproof frying pan. Add green onion and cook for 4-5 mins until softened.
3. Stir in the garlic and chilli, and cook for a couple mins more.
4. Add the 1/2 cup water. Season well and stir through the ready-roasted peppers and ham. Bring to a simmer and cook for 10 mins.
5. Add the kale, stirring through to wilt.
6. In a small bowl, beat the eggs with a pinch of cayenne and pour in frying pan together with other ingredients.
7. Transfer the frying pan to the oven and bake for 10 mins.
8. Serve hot.

Servings: 2

Cooking Times

Preparation Time: 10 minutes

Cooking Time: 30 minutes

Total Time: 2 hours and 20 minutes

Nutrition Facts (per serving)

Total Carbohydrates: 3,8g

Dietary Fiber: 0,8g

Net Carbs: 0,5g

Protein: 22g

Total Fat: 15,74g

Calories: 251

Bell Pepper and Ham Omelet

Ingredients

4 large eggs

1 cup green pepper (chopped)

1/4 lb ham, cooked and diced

1 green onion, diced

1 tsp coconut oil

salt and freshly ground pepper to taste

Directions

1. Wash and chop vegetables. Set aside.
2. Into a small bowl beat the eggs. Set aside.
3. Heat non-stick skillet over medium heat and add coconut oil. Pour half of the beaten eggs into the skillet.
4. When the egg has partially set, add half of the vegetables and ham to one half of the omelet and continue to cook until the egg is almost fully set.
5. Fold the empty half over top of the ham and veggies using a spatula.
6. Cook for 2 minutes more and then serve.
7. Serve hot.

Servings: 2

Nutrition Facts (per serving)

Total Carbohydrates: 6,8g

Protein: 21,88g

Total Fat: 12g

Calories: 225,76

Chia Flour Pancakes

Ingredients

1 cup Chia flour

2 tsp sweetener of your choice

1 egg, beaten

1 Tbsp coconut butter or oil

1/2 cup coconut milk (canned)

Directions

1. In a medium bowl, combine the flour and sugar. Add the egg, milk and coconut butter. Mix well until make a smooth batter.
2. Grease a non-stick skillet and heat over medium-high heat. Drop a heaping tablespoon of batter onto the hot surface.
3. When bubbles form on the surface of the scones, use a spatula to turn them and then cook about 2 minutes per side.
4. Serve hot.

Servings: 6

Cooking Time: 15 minutes

Nutrition Facts (per serving)

Total Carbohydrates: 4,65g

Net Carbs: 2,54g

Protein: 2,46g

Total Fat: 3,5g

Calories: 59

Choco Moko Chia Porridge

Ingredients

3 Tbs Chia Seeds

1 cup almond milk, unsweetened

2 tsp cocoa powder

1/4 cup raspberries -fresh or frozen

2 Tbsp almond, ground

Sweetener of your choice (optional)

Directions

1. Mix and stir the almond milk and the cocoa powder together.
2. Add the Chia Seeds in the mixture.
3. Mix well with a fork.
4. Place the mixture in a fridge for 30 minutes.
5. Serve with raspberries and ground almonds on the top. (optional)

Servings: 2

Inactive Time: 30 minutes. Cooking Time: 5 minutes

Nutrition Facts (per serving)

Total Carbohydrates: 15,2g

Dietary Fiber: 11,28g

Net Carbs: 1g

Protein: 5,47g

Total Fat: 9,62g

Calories: 150,15

Coffee Flaxseed Dream Breakfast

Ingredients

3 Tbsp flaxseed, ground

1/2 cup strong black coffee, unsweetened

2 1/2 Tbsp coconut flakes, unsweetened

1 Tbsp coconut oil, melted

Sweetener of your choice to taste

1/2 cup water (optional)

Directions

1. In a bowl, combine the flaxseed and the coconut flakes.
2. Add the melted coconut oil, then pour the hot coffee over it and mix.
3. If it is too thick, add a little water.
4. At the end, add the sweetener of your choice to taste.
5. Ready! Enjoy!!

Servings: 1

Nutrition Facts (per serving)

Total Carbohydrates: 1,52

Dietary Fiber: 0,9g

Net Carbs: 0,62g

Protein: 1,48g

Total Fat: 22,1

Calories: 246,43

Crimini Mushroom with Boiled Eggs Breakfast

Ingredients

14 Crimini mushroom, finely chopped

8 large eggs, hard-boiled, chopped

6 slices bacon or pancetta

1 spring onion, diced

Salt and ground black pepper to taste

Directions

1. In a frying pan cook bacon. Reserve a bacon fat in the pan. Chop up bacon pieces and set aside.
2. In a deep saucepan, hard-boil the eggs. When ready, wah, clean, shell and chop into bite-size pieces.
3. In a frying pan cook the spring onion with remaining bacon fat over medium-high heat.
4. Add the Crimini mushrooms and sauté another 5-6 minutes.
5. Blend the eggs, bacon and cook together. Adjust salt and ground black pepper to taste.
6. Serve.

Servings: 6

Cooking Time: 20 minutes

Nutrition Facts (per serving)

Total Carbohydrates: 2,43g

Dietary Fiber: 1,5g

Protein: 11,32

Total Fat: 13,38

Calories: 176,15

Egg Whites and Spinach Omelet

Ingredients

5 egg whites

2 Tbsp almond milk

1 zucchini, shredded

1 cup spinach leaves, fresh

2 Tbs spring onion, chopped

2 cloves garlic

Olive oil

Basil leaves, fresh, chopped

Salt and ground black pepper to taste

Directions

1. Wash and chop the vegetables
2. In a bowl, beat the egg whites and the almond milk.
3. In a greased frying pan with olive oil, cook the vegetables (spinach, zucchini, spring onion) just for one to two minutes.
4. Put the vegetables on the side, grease the pan again with olive oil and pour the eggs. Cook until the eggs are firm. Add the vegetables on one side and cook for two minutes more. Adjust salt and pepper to taste.
5. Decorate with basil leaves and serve.

Servings: 2

Cooking Times

Total Time: 15 minutes

Nutrition Facts (per serving)

Total Carbohydrates: 5,78g

Dietary Fiber: 1,58g

Net Carbs: 3,4g

Protein: 11,08g

Total Fat: 1,56g

Calories: 70,8

Fast Protein and Peanut-Butter Pancakes

Ingredients

1 scoop of low-carb protein powder

2 eggs

2 Tbsp of natural peanut butter

2 Tbsp flaxseed

2 Tbsp water

olive oil for greasing

Instructions

1. In a bowl, mix protein powder, eggs, peanut butter, water and flaxseeds.
2. Grease with olive oil and heat a large non-stick frying pan over medium heat.
3. Laddle a batter mixture and cook for 2 minutes per side or until bubbles appear on surface. Transfer to a plate.
4. Serve hot.

Servings: 1

Cooking Time: 15 minutes

Nutrition Facts (per serving)

Total Carbohydrates: 13,78g

Dietary Fiber: 8,48g

Protein: 17,8g

Total Fat: 23,59g

Calories: 406,41

Guacamole Bacon and Eggs Breakfast

Ingredients

4 slices bacon or pancetta

2 Tbsp heavy cream

2 Tbsp avocado oil

4 eggs

salt and peppet to taste

Directions

1. In a bowl, beat eggs with heavy cream and salt and ground pepper to taste.
2. Pour egg mixture over bacon and cook for 2-3 minutes.
3. Flip bacon and eggs on other side and cook for 1 minute more.
4. Serve and enjoy!

Servings: 4

Cooking Time: 13 minutes

Nutrition Facts (per serving)

Total Carbohydrates: 0,66g

Dietary Fiber: 0g

Net Carbs: 0,15g

Protein: 9,28g

Total Fat: 22,43g

Calories: 292

Hemp Muffins with Walnuts

Ingredients

2 1/2 cup Hemp flour

1 1/2 cup walnuts, chopped

1/2 cup sweetener of your choice

4 Tbsp extra-virgin olive oil

1 tsp vanilla extract

2 tsp baking powder

1 tsp baking soda

Directions

1. Preheat oven to 345F.
2. In a small bowl whisk olive oil, sweetener of your choice and vanilla.
3. In a separate bowl, combine hemp flour, baking powder and baking soda. Add in chopped walnuts and toss to coat.
4. Add olive oil mixture to the flour mixture and stir slightly.
5. Spoon a batter into 12 muffin cups, filling 3/4 full.
6. Bake 18 - 20 minutes. Allow to cool 10 minutes in the muffin pan, then turn out onto a wire rack to cool completely. Serve.

Servings: 12

Cooking Time: 30 minutes

Nutrition Facts (per serving)

Total Carbohydrates: 25,18g

Dietary Fiber: 4,43g

Net Carbs: 1,68g

Protein: 7,75g

Total Fat: 16,45g

Calories: 270,41

Baked Pancetta and Eggs

Ingredients

6 slices Pancetta, crumbled

8 eggs

3/4 cup Cheddar cheese, grated

3/4 cup heavy cream

salt and pepper to taste

olive oil for greasing

Directions

1. Preheat the oven to 350 degrees F. Grease a big baking dish with olive oil.
2. In a bowl, beat the eggs with shredded Cheddar cheese and cream, and season with salt and pepper to taste.
3. Crumble Pancetta evenly over the egg mixture. Put the baking dish in a preheated oven.
4. Bake for 15 minutes.
5. Serve immediately.

Servings: 6

Cooking Times: 20 minutes

Nutrition Facts (per serving)

Total Carbohydrates: 1,49g

Dietary Fiber: 0g

Protein: 12,5g

Total Fat: 22,03g

Calories: 254,89

Bilberry Coconut Mush

Ingredients

1/4 cup coconut flour

1 cup coconut milk

1/4 cup ground flaxseed

1 tsp vanilla extract

1 tsp cinnamon

Liquid sweetener of your choice

Toppings

1 cup bilberries

2 Tbs shaved coconut

2 Tbs pumpkin seeds

Directions

1. In a saucepan heat the coconut milk. Add in coconut flour, cinnamon and flaxseed and whisk.
2. Add in vanilla extract and liquid sweetener of your choice. Cook for 10 minutes stirring constantly. Remove from heat and let cook for 2-3 minutes.
3. Decorate with fresh bilberries, pumpkin seeds and shaved coconut to taste.

Servings: 2

Cooking Times

Total Time: 5 minutes

Nutrition Facts (per serving)

Total Carbohydrates: 16,4g

Dietary Fiber: 1,69

Net Carbs: 4,76g

Protein: 2,86g

Total Fat: 22,4f

Calories:445

Boiled Eggs with Mascarpone and Bacon

Ingredients

2 large eggs

2 Tbsp Mascarpone cheese

2 Tbs crumbled bacon

1 Tbs coconut butter

salt and pepper to taste

Directions

1. Hard boil the eggs; bring water to a boil over medium-high heat, then cover, remove from the heat and set aside for 10 minutes.
2. Wash, peel and chop boiled eggs and place them in a large bowl.
3. Add the butter and the Mascarpone cheese, mix well. Adjust salt and pepper to taste.
4. Serve.

Servings: 2

Cooking Time: 15 minutes

Nutrition Facts (per serving)

Total Carbohydrates: 0,91g

Dietary Fiber: 0g

Net Carbs: 0,19g

Protein: 11,1g

Total Fat: 22,84g

Calories: 328,34

Flax-Almond Coated Cheddar

Ingredients

4 oz Cheddar cheese, 2 slices

1 large egg

1 tsp almond flour or ground almonds

1 Tbsp flaxseed, ground

1 tsp hemp seeds

1 Tbsp Olive oil

Salt and pepper to taste

Directions

1. In a non-stick frying pan heat a tablespoon of olive oil.
2. In a bowl, combine the almond flour, the ground flaxseed and the hemp seeds.
3. In a separate bowl, beat an egg together with the salt and pepper.
4. Coat the cheddar slices first with the egg mix and then with the dry mix. Fry cheese for about 3 minutes on each side. Serve hot.

Servings: 2

Cooking Time: 15 minutes

Nutrition Facts (per serving)

Total Carbohydrates: 4,28g

Dietary Fiber: 2,83g

Protein: 17,91g

Total Fat: 22,37g

Calories: 358,62

French Almond Toast

Ingredients

4 eggs

1/4 cup coconut milk

2 Tbsp coconut oil (melted)

6 slices almond bread

2 tsp sweetener of your choice (optional)

1/2 tsp cinnamon powder

1 tsp organic vanilla extract

salt and pepper (per taste)

Directions

1. Whisk coconut milk, sweetener of your choice, eggs, organic vanilla extract, salt and cinnamon.
2. Soak each slice of almond bread (or any gluten free vegan Hemp & Seed bread) in egg mixture.
3. In a frying pan, heat the coconut oil over high heat; cook each slice of bread three minutes or until golden. Transfer toast to the plate lined with paper.
4. Serve hot.

Servings: 6

Nutrition Facts (per serving)

Total Carbohydrates: 11,13g

Dietary Fiber: 0,57g

Protein: 6,56g

Total Fat: 10,2g

Calories: 162,6

Pork and Sage Breakfast Burgers

Ingredients

1 lb ground pork

2 Tbsp fresh sage, chopped

1 tsp garlic powder

1 tsp cayenne pepper

salt and pepper to taste

2 Tbsp granular sweetener of your choice

olive oil for greasing

Directions

1. In a large bowl, combine all ingredients except olive oil. Use hands to mix thoroughly.
2. Form into 8 evenly burgers.
3. Grease with olive oil your large frying pan over medium heat.
4. Add burger and cook about 3 to 4 minutes per side.
5. Ready. Serve and enjoy!!

Servings: 4

Cooking Time: 15 minutes

Nutrition Facts (per serving)

Total Carbohydrates: 0,78g

Dietary Fiber: 0,44g

Net Carbs: 0,03g

Protein: 19,29g

Total Fat: 22,17g

Calories: 302,21

Quick & Easy Flax "Muffins"

Ingredients

4 Tbsp ground flax meal

1 egg

1 Tbs of heavy whipping cream

1 tsp organic vanilla extract

2 tsp sweetener of your choice

1 pinch salt

coconut butter

cocoa powder (optional)

Directions

1. Mix all ingredients in a microwave safe bowl; stir to combine well.
2. Place a bit of coconut butter on the top. Microwave for one and a half minutes.
3. If you want, you can add a splash of unsweetened cocoa powder.
4. Ready! Serve! Enjoy!

Servings: 1

Cooking Times

Total Time: 5 minutes

Nutrition Facts (per serving)

Total Carbohydrates: 10,24g

Dietary Fiber: 1,36g

Net Carbs: 0,86g

Protein: 8,21g

Total Fat: 8,4g

Calories: 160,51

Millet Gingerbread Mash

Ingredients

1 cup millet flour (or any kind of whole grain flour)

4 cups water

1/2 tsp ground ginger

1/4 tsp ground allspice

1/8 tsp ground nutmeg

1/4 tsp ground cardamom

1/4 tsp ground coriander

1 1/2 Tbs ground cinnamon

1 tsp ground cloves

sweetener of your choice (optional)

Directions

1. In a medium saucepan bring water to boiling and cook the millet flour to package direction. Add in all spices together and stir.
2. Reduce heat and simmer, uncovered, for 5 minutes, stirring occasionally.
3. When cooked, add sweetener to taste.

Servings: 6

Nutrition Facts (per serving)

Total Carbohydrates: 11,13g

Dietary Fiber: 2,6g

Protein: 1,9g

Total Fat: 2.82g

Calories: 58,18

Scrambled Eggs with Bacon and Gouda Cheese

Ingredients

4 strips cooked bacon

4 eggs

2 1/2 Tbsp olive oil

1/4 cup softened cream cheese

1/4 cup shredded Gouda cheese

garlic and onion powder

black or white pepper

Directions

1. In a frying pan heat some olive oil and fry bacon slices until crisp .
2. In a small bowl beat the eggs with onion and garlic powder, cream cheese and Gouda shredded cheese. Season with salt and pepper to taste.
3. Pour egg mixture over bacon slices and cook for 3-4 minutes. Serve and enjoy!

Servings: 4

Cooking Time: 15 minutes

Nutrition Facts (per serving)

Total Carbohydrates: 1,47g

Dietary Fiber: 0g

Protein: 14,44g

Total Fat: 25,94g

Calories: 380,72

Beet Cucumber Smoothie

Ingredients

1 cup spinach leaves

2 cups cucumber (peeled, seeded and chopped)

1/2 cup carrot chopped

1/2 cup fresh beetroot

3/4 cup heavy (whipping) cream

4 tsp sweetener of your choice (optional)

Handful of ground almonds

1 cup ice cubes

1 cup water

Directions

1. Place all ingredients in a blender.
2. Pulse until smooth.
3. Serve immediately.

Servings: 4

Cooking Time: 5 minutes

Nutrition Facts (per serving)

Total Carbohydrates: 6,19g

Protein: 1,66g

Total Fat: 12.99g

Calories: 137,91

Cilantro and Ginger Smoothie

Ingredients

1/2 cup fresh cilantro (chopped)

2 inch ginger, fresh

1 cucumber

2 Tbsp chia seeds

1/2 cup spinach, fresh

1 Tbsp almond butter

Handful of ground almond

1 lime (or lemon)

2 cups water

Directions

1. Blend spinach, coriander and water until smooth.
2. Add the remaining fruits and blend again.

Servings: 3

Cooking Time: 5 minutes

Nutrition Facts (per serving)

Total Carbohydrates: 11,98g

Dietary Fiber: 6,88g

Net Carbs: 13,96g,71g

Protein:

Total Fat: 6.92g

Calories: 102,72

Green Coconut Smoothie

Ingredients

1 cup coconut milk

1 green apple, cored and chopped

1 cup spinach

1 cucumber

2 Tbsp shaved coconut

1/2 cup water

ice cubes (if needed)

Directions

1. Put all ingredients and ice in a blender; pulse until smooth.
2. Serve immediately.

Servings: 2

Cooking Time: 5 minutes

Nutrition Facts (per serving)

Total Carbohydrates: 18,11g

Dietary Fiber: 4g

Net Carbs: 8,79g

Protein: 2,88g

Total Fat: 16,56g

Calories: 216,57

Green Devil Smoothie

Ingredients

3 cup kale, fresh

1/2 cup coconut yogurt

1/2 cup broccoli, florets

2 celery stalk, chopped

2 cup water

1 Tbsp lemon juice

ice cubes (if needed)

Directions

1. Blend all ingredients together until smooth and slightly frothy.

Servings: 2

Cooking Time: 10 minutes

Nutrition Facts (per serving)

Total Carbohydrates: 16,42g

Dietary Fiber: 6,18g

Net Carbs: 1,89g

Protein: 4,09g

Total Fat: 4,98g

Calories: 117,09

Green Dream Smoothie

Ingredients

1 cup raw cucumber, peeled and sliced

4 cups water

1 cup romaine lettuce

1 cup Haas avocado

2 Tbsp fresh basil

sweetener of your choice (optional)

handful of walnuts

2 Tbsp fresh parsley

1 Tbsp fresh ginger grated

ice cubes (optional)

Directions

1. In a blender, combine all of the ingredients and puls until smooth.
2. Add ice if used. Serve cold.

Servings: 4

Nutrition Facts (per serving)

Total Carbohydrates: 4,1g

Net Carbs: 1,07g

Protein: 1,1g

Total Fat: 3,89g

Calories: 50,62

Green Pistachio Smoothie

Ingredients

2 celery stem with leaves

1 cup spinach leaves, roughly chopped

1/2 cup pistachio nuts (unsalted)

1/2 avocado, chopped

1/2 cup lime, juice

1 Tbsp Hemp seeds

1 Tbsp soaked almonds

1 cup coconut water or water

ice cubes (optional)

Directions

1. Mix all ingredients in a blender with a few ice cubes until smooth.

Servings: 2

Cooking Time: 10 minutes

Nutrition Facts (per serving)

Total Carbohydrates: 14,4g

Dietary Fiber: 9,8g

Net Carbs: 5,01

Protein: 11,08g

Total Fat: 17,88g

Calories: 349,55

Lime Peppermint Smoothie

Ingredients

1/4 cup fresh mint leaves

1/4 cup lime juice

1/2 cup cucumber, chopped

1 Tbsp fresh basil leaves, chopped

1 tsp chia seed (optional)

Handful of chia seeds

3 tsp zest of limes

sweetener of your choice to taste

1 cup water, divided

Ice as needed

Directions

1. Place all ingredients in a blender or food processor. Pulse until smooth well.
2. Fill glasses with ice, pour the limeade into each glass, and enjoy!

Servings: 4

Cooking Times

Total Time: 5 minutes

Nutrition Facts (per serving)

Total Carbohydrates: 4,49g

Dietary Fiber: 1,98g

Net Carbs: 0,75g

Protein: 0,84g

Total Fat: 1,16g

Calories: 28,11

Red Grapefruit Kale Smoothies

Ingredients

2 cups Cantaloupe

1/4 cup fresh strawberries

8 oz coconut yogurt

2 cups kale leaves, chopped

2 Tbsp sweetener of your taste

1 Ice as needed

1 cup water

Directions

1. Clean the grapefruit and remove the seeds.
2. Combine all ingredients in an electric blender and whirl until smooth. Add ice if used and serve.

Servings: 4

Cooking Time: 10 minutes

Nutrition Facts (per serving)

Total Carbohydrates: 14g

Dietary Fiber: 7,23g

Net Carbs: 2,96g

Protein: 4,42g

Total Fat: 11,57g

Calories: 260,74

Simple Avocado Smoothie

Ingredients

2.6 oz avocado

2 cup water

2 tsp chia seeds

0.5 oz fresh spinach

2 fl oz heavy whipping cream

1 tsp vanilla extract, unsweetened

1 Tbsp extra virgin coconut oil

liquid Stevia extract

few ice cubes

Directions

1. First, bisect the avocado. Carefully remove the seed.
2. In a blender, put all ingredients, sweetener and the ice (if used) and beat until smooth. Serve.

Servings: 2

Cooking Time: 10 minutes

Nutrition Facts (per serving)

Total Carbohydrates: 4,46g

Net Carbs: 0,18g

Protein: 1,66g

Total Fat: 23,63g

Calories: 226,44

Vanilla Protein Smoothie

Ingredients

1 cup baby spinach

5 Tbsp of heavy cream

3 Tbsp organic nut butter of your choice

1/2 cup vanilla protein powder

3 Tbsp sweetener of your choice

1 cup of water

Ice cubes

Directions

1. Place all ingredients in a blender and pulse until smooth well.
2. Serve with ice cubes (optional).

Servings: 2

Cooking Time: 5 minutes

Nutrition Facts (per serving)

Total Carbohydrates: 11,88g

Dietary Fiber: 4,63g

Net Carbs: 3,88g

Protein: 8,41g

Total Fat: 21,79g

Calories: 256,18

Ail Creamy Brussels Sprouts

Ingredients

10 Brussels sprouts

4 cloves garlic

1/4 cup cream cheese

2 Tbsp extra virgin olive oil

1 tsp Balsamic vinegar

salt and pepper to taste

Directions

1. Clean the Brussels Sprouts discarding the first leaves and cut into julienne strips.
2. Peel and chop the garlic cloves.
3. In a frying pan, heat the olive oil and saute the Brussels Sprouts and garlic,
4. When the garlic and sprouts are tender, turn off the heat and add the cheese. Let sit for a couple of minutes.
5. Transfer to plate and enjoy!

Servings: 1

Cooking Time: 15 minutes

Nutrition Facts (per serving)

Total Carbohydrates: 16,99g

Dietary Fiber: 6,22g

Net Carbs: 5,21g

Protein: 9,27g

Total Fat: 12,55g

Calories: 223,26

Baked Broccoli with Mushrooms and Parmesan

Ingredients

4 cups broccoli

2 cups mushrooms (chopped fine)

2 Tbsp minced garlic

1/2 tsp dried oregano

3 Tbsp grated Parmesan

salt and ground black pepper to taste

Directions

1. Preheat oven to 300F. Line a baking sheet with parchment paper.
2. Wash and slice broccoli into florets. In a bowl, toss broccoli and finely chopped mushrooms in olive oil. Season with dried oregano, salt and pepper to taste.
3. Spread all vegetables evenly over the prepared baking pan. Bake for 20-25 minutes until the broccoli is browned.
4. When done, leave to cool 5 minutes, sprinkle with Parmesan cheese and serve.

Servings: 2

Cooking Times

Total Time: 35 minutes

Nutrition Facts (per serving)

Total Carbohydrates: 16,22g

Dietary Fiber: 3,33g

Net Carbs: 4,86g

Protein: 12,16g

Total Fat: 3,51g

Calories: 138,26

Baked Buckwheat Pancakes with Hazelnuts

Ingredients

1/2 cup buckwheat flour

3 eggs

1/2 cup coconut cream

1 vanilla bean (seeds only)

1 pinch of salt

3 Tbsp olive oil

Liquid sweetener of your choice

hazelnuts

Directions

1. Preheat oven to 400F degrees.
2. Grease an oval baking pan.
3. In a large bowl, add eggs, milk, flour, vanilla and salt. Mix the ingredients until the mixture become homogeneous.
4. Pour batter in prepared oval baking pan evenly. Bake for 15-20 minutes.
5. Remove the pancake from the pan and serve with sweetener of your taste and hazelnuts.

Servings: 2

Cooking Times

Total Time: 30 minutes

Nutrition Facts (per serving)

Total Carbohydrates: 17,46g

Dietary Fiber: 3g

Net Carbs: 3,16g

Protein: 14,4g

Total Fat: 22,66g

Calories: 390,07

Baked Parmesan-Almond Zucchini

Ingredients

2 zucchinis, thinly sliced to about 1-inch thick rounds

3 large eggs, beaten

1 cup almond flour

1 cup almonds, ground

1 cup grated Parmesan cheese

1 tsp dried oregano

salt and pepper

Directions

1. Preheat oven to 400 F degrees. Line a large baking sheet with parchment paper.
2. Wash, clean and slice zucchinis. Salt from all sides and let dry on a paper towel. Set aside.
3. In a plate, combine ground almond, Parmesan cheese, oregano and season with salt and pepper to taste and oregano; set aside.
4. In another shallow plate add the almond flour.
5. In a third plate beat eggs, with salt and pepper.
6. Start dredging zucchini rounds in flour, dip into eggs, then dredge in almond mixture, pressing to coat. Place zucchini slices on prepared baking sheet.
7. Bake for 20 to 30 minutes, or until the zucchini rounds are golden and crispy.
8. Serve hot.

Servings: 6

Cooking Times

Preparation Time: 15 minutes

Cooking Time: 25 minutes

Total Time: 40 minutes

Nutrition Facts (per serving)

Total Carbohydrates: 16,36g

Dietary Fiber: 3,28g

Net Carbs: 3,16g

Protein: 12,12g

Total Fat: 17,49g

Calories: 288,89

Double Cheese Artichoke Dip

Ingredients

2 cup artichoke hearts, chopped

16 oz shredded Mozzarella cheese

1 cup grated Parmesan cheese

1 cup heavy (whipping) cream

1 cup green onion, grated

Directions

1. Mix all ingredients together and put in a Slow Cooker.
2. Cook on HIGH mode for about one hour.
3. Sprinkle with chopped green onion, if desired.

Servings: 12

Cooking Times

Total Time: 1 hour

Nutrition Facts (per serving)

Total Carbohydrates: 10,44g

Dietary Fiber: 1,74g

Net Carbs: 2,32g

Protein: 13,67g

Total Fat: 15g

Calories: 227,64

Easy Slow Cooker Artichokes

Ingredients

4 artichokes

3 Tbsp lemon juice

2 Tbsp coconut butter, melted

1 tsp salt and ground black pepper to taste

water

Directions

1. Wash and trim artichokes.
2. Start by pulling off the outermost leaves until you get down to the lighter yellow leaves.
3. Then, using a serrated knife, cut off the top third or so of the artichoke.
4. With the same serrated knife, trim the very bottom of the stem.
5. Mix together salt, melted coconut butter and lemon juice and pour over artichokes.
6. Pour in water to cover 3 of artichokes. Cover and cook on LOW 8-10 hours or on HIGH 2-4 hours.
7. Serve and enjoy!

Servings: 4

Cooking Times

Total Time: 2 hours and 10 minutes

Nutrition Facts (per serving)

Total Carbohydrates: 14,52g

Dietary Fiber: 6,95g

Net Carbs: 1,56g

Protein: 4,29g

Total Fat: 6,98g

Calories: 113,58

Eggs with Motley Peppers and Zucchini

Ingredients

6 eggs

2 zucchini, diced

1 spring onion, chopped

1 green pepper, finely diced

1 yellow pepper, finely diced

1 red pepper, finely diced

3 Tbsp coconut oil (melted)

salt and fresh ground black pepper to taste

Directions

1. In a non-stick frying skillet, heat 2 Tbsp olive oil in a pan and sauté the onion for 5 minutes.
2. Add the peppers and fry for 2-3 minutes more.
3. Next, add the zucchini and sauté for another 3 minutes. Remove from heat and set aside.
4. In a medium bowl beat the eggs with salt.
5. Mix the vegetables into the eggs.
6. Heat the remaining olive oil in the frying pan and pour in the egg and vegetable mixture.
7. Cook for 2-3 minutes constantly stirring.
8. Serve hot.

Servings: 4

Cooking Times

Total Time: 25 minutes

Nutrition Facts (per serving)

Total Carbohydrates: 12,77g

Dietary Fiber: 3,26g

Net Carbs: 6,55g

Protein: 12,04g

Total Fat: 7.94g

Calories: 165,31

Electric Pressure Cooker Bok Choy Salad

Ingredients

1 bunch bok choi, trimmed

1 cup or more water

Salt

Olive oil

Lime

Directions

1. Place the stems in your Electric pressure cooker and pour one cup, or more water to just-cover the stems.
2. Close and lock the lid of the pressure cooker. Turn the heat up to high and when the cooker reaches pressure, lower to the heat to the minimum required by the cooker to maintain pressure.
3. Cook for 5-7 minutes at high pressure.
4. When time is up, open the cooker by Slow releasing the pressure.
5. Pull out the leaves and stems with tongs, and put on a small serving plate.
6. Dress with salt and olive oil before serving. Sprinkle some lime juice.

Servings: 3

Cooking Times

Total Time: 10 minutes

Nutrition Facts (per serving)

Total Carbohydrates: 6,1g

Dietary Fiber: 2,8g

Net Carbs: 3,1g

Protein: 4,2g

Total Fat: 0,56g

Calories: 36,4

Kale, Peppers and Crumbled Feta Omelet (Slow Cooker)

Ingredients

8 eggs, well beaten

1 cup red peppers, diced

1/4 cup green onions (finely chopped)

1/2 cup crumbled Feta

3/4 cup kale, chopped

2 tsp olive oil

1/2 tsp Italian seasoning

Salt and freshly ground pepper, to taste

sour cream cheese or cottage (optional)

Directions

1. In a large frying pan heat oil on medium-high. Add chopped kale and cook about 3-4 minutes.
2. Wash and chop the red peppers. Slice the green onions and crumble the Feta. Grease the bottom of your Slow Cooker with olive oil. Add the chopped red pepper and sliced green onion to Slow Cooker with the kale.
3. In a small bowl, beat the eggs and pour over other ingredients in Slow Cooker. Stir well and add Italian seasonings. Adjust salt and pepper to taste.
4. Cook on LOW for 2 - 3 hours. Serve hot, with a dollop of sour cream if desired.

Servings: 4

Cooking Times

Total Time: 3 hours

Nutrition Facts (per serving)

Total Carbohydrates: 4,56g

Dietary Fiber: 1,01g

Net Carbs: 1,16g

Protein: 11,78g

Total Fat: 23,87g

Calories: 279,34

Low Carb Almond Buns

Ingredients

3 almond flour

5 Tbs butter, unsalted

2 eggs

1.5 tsp sweetener of your choice (optional)

1.5 tsp baking powder

Directions

1. Preheat oven to 350F.
2. Combine the dry ingredients in a bowl.
3. In a separate bowl, whisk the eggs.
4. Melt butter, add to mixture and whisk well.
5. Divide mixture equally into 6 parts and place in a greased baking dish.
6. Bake for 12-15 minutes.
7. Let cool on a wire rack.

Servings: 3

Cooking Time: 20 minutes

Nutrition Facts (per serving)

Total Carbohydrates: 2,44g

Dietary Fiber: 0,2g

Net Carbs: 1,22g

Protein: 4,45g

Total Fat: 22,43g

Calories: 225,58

Mini Ham Omelets Muffins

Ingredients

11 oz Ham Steak

10 green onions Green Onions

12 Eggs

1/2 cup of Heavy cream

9 slices mushrooms

9 Slices Cheddar Cheese

coconut oil for greasing

Salt, Pepper, Onion Powder, Garlic Powder to taste

Directions

1. Preheat oven to 350F. Grease the muffin pan with coconut oil.
2. Dice the ham steak, slice the green onions and wash the mushrooms.
3. In a deep bowl, beat the eggs. Add in the heavy cream and spices along with ham cubes and sliced green onions.
4. Adjust salt, pepper and spices to taste.
5. Fill each cavity of muffin pan with the egg mixture.
6. Bake in oven for 4-5 minutes.
7. Remove from the oven and add the mushrooms on the top
8. Cook for 8-9 more minutes or until the eggs are mostly set.
9. Add Cheddar cheese and cook for 1 more minute.
10. Serve hot.

Servings: 18

Cooking Times

Total Time: 25 minutes

Nutrition Facts (per serving)

Total Carbohydrates: 1,54g

Dietary Fiber: 0,32g

Net Carbs: 0,59g

Protein: 11,69g

Total Fat: 11,1g

Calories: 153,55

Nonpareil Bacon Waffles

Ingredients

4 slices bacon

2 eggs

3 cup almond flour

5 Tbsp melted butter or ghee

1.5 tsp baking powder

1.5 tsp sweetener of your choice

Directions

1. Microwave the butter and set aside.
2. In a frying pan, cook the bacon until crisp.
3. First, mix the dry ingredients first (almond flour, baking powder and sweetener of your choice)
4. Add the two eggs and mix thoroughly. Add the melted butter and mix.
5. Preheat the waffle maker.
6. When it is preheated, open it, fill with batter and place 2 slices of bacon over top.
7. Close and flip the waffle maker, when it beeps, flip it over and remove the waffle with a fork.
8. Serve hot.

Servings: 2

Cooking Times

Total Time: 15 minutes

Nutrition Facts (per serving)

Total Carbohydrates: 5,1g

Dietary Fiber: 2,65g

Net Carbs: 1,89g

Protein: 8,35g

Total Fat: 24,97g

Calories: 323,24

Power Greens and Sausage Casserole

Ingredients

12 eggs

1 1/4 lbs chicken or turkey sausage

1 cup kale leaves, chopped

1 cup arugula leaves, chopped

2 cups spinach, finely chopped

2 small zucchini - peeled

1 green onion, chopped

1/4 cup coconut milk

1/2 Tbsp coconut oil

1 tsp garlic powder

1 tsp sea salt

1 tsp pepper

Directions

1. Heat oven to 365 degrees. Grease casserole dish with coconut oil.
2. In a frying pan, melt coconut oil over medium heat, Add in sausage and stir with a wooden spoon. Cook for two to three minutes.
3. In a big bowl beat eggs.
4. Chop the green onion and peeled the zucchini. Mix into eggs with seasoning, all greens and coconut milk.
5. Pour in egg mixture and stir in sausage. Adjust the salt and pepper to taste. Cook for 45 minutes.
6. Cover with foil and cook for 10-15 minutes more.
   7. Serve hot.

Servings: 10

Cooking Times

Total Time: 20 minutes

Nutrition Facts (per serving)

Total Carbohydrates: 11,88g

Dietary Fiber: 1,48g

Net Carbs: 1,81

Protein: 12,19g

Total Fat: 7,98g

Calories: 165,48

Radish, Bacon and Egg Scramble

Ingredients

6 oz radishes

4 oz Cheddar cheese

8 oz flank steak

2 oz bacon

4 eggs

Salt and Pepper to taste

Directions

1. Preheat oven to 450 degrees F. Wash the radishes, then cut the ends and quarter. Set aside.
2. In a frying pan, cook the flank steak for 5 minutes flipping from one side to another.
3. Pan fry the radishes and bacon in a cast iron skillet for about 5-6 minutes or until the radishes turn golden brown
4. Slice the flank steak and add into the pan.
5. Add the cheese and break the eggs into the mixture, season to taste and cook for one to two minutes.
6. Transfer to the oven and cook for 12 minutes until the eggs are set to the desired leve.
7. Serve and enjoy!

Servings: 4

Cooking Times

Total Time: 25 minutes

Nutrition Facts (per serving)

Total Carbohydrates: 2,26g

Dietary Fiber: 0,68g

Net Carbs: 1,12g

Protein: 27,42g

Total Fat: 22,04g

Calories: 348,58

Sautéed Cabbage and Brussels Sprouts (Electric Pressure Cooker)

Ingredients

4 medium beets

1-1/2 lbs cabbage, cut into wedges

1-1/2 lbs Brussels sprouts

8 large cloves garlic, left unpeeled

3 Tbsp olive oil

1 Tbsp chopped fresh thyme

1/2 tsp salt, plus more to taste

1/4 tsp freshly ground black pepper

Directions

1. In your Electric Pressure Cooker add chopped vegetables, oil, salt and freshly ground black pepper.
2. Select SAUTE and cook under HIGH pressure for 15 minutes.
3. When ready, select natural release. Carefully open the lid.
4. Transfer all vegetables from the cooker to the serving plate, toss well and serve.

Servings: 6

Cooking Times

Total Time: 15 minutes

Nutrition Facts (per serving)

Total Carbohydrates: 16,11g

Dietary Fiber: 6,57g

Net Carbs: 7,82g

Protein: 6,2g

Total Fat: 8,31g

Calories: 160,91

Simple Bacon Pepper Pot

Ingredients

6 slices bacon

4 Eggs

1 small green pepper

Jalapeno pepper, sliced

1 green onion

Directions

1. Slice the pepper, green onion and jalapeno into thin strips.
2. In a frying pan, cook the vegetables about 2-3 minutes until browned.
3. Chop the bacon in a food processor until it breaks into chunks.
4. Mix all the ingredients together.
5. Cook the hash until the bacon is approaching crisp.
6. Arrange on a plate and top with a fried egg!
7. Serve and enjoy!

Servings: 2

Cooking Time: 25 minutes

Nutrition Facts (per serving)

Total Carbohydrates: 4,41g

Dietary Fiber: 1,44g

Net Carbs: 2,29g

Protein: 23,33g

Total Fat: 29,87g

Calories: 499,69

Sour and Spicy Goat Skewers

Ingredients

1 lb boneless goat loin, cut into cubes

2 Tbsp lime juice (freshly squeezed)

1 cup coconut yogurt

1/4 tsp ground ginger

3/4 tsp turmeric

1/2 tsp ground cumin

1 Tbs ground coriander

1/2 tsp salt

Skewers

Directions

1. In a medium bowl, stir together coconut yogurt, lime juice and all seasonings; mix well.
2. Add the goat meat cubes to the bowl, stir to coat with the marinade, cover and refrigerate for 6-8 hours.
3. Remove the meat from the marinade, pat lightly with paper towels to dry.
4. Place meat evenly on the skewers. Grill over medium-hot coals, turning frequently, for about 10 minutes until nicely brown.
5. Serve and enjoy without guilty.

Servings: 2

Cooking Times

Inactive Time: 10 minutes

Total Time: 25 minutes

Nutrition Facts (per serving)

Total Carbohydrates: 12,24g

Dietary Fiber: 1,25g

Net Carbs: 7,96g

Protein: 26,77g

Total Fat: 9,79g

Calories: 342,93

Sour Sausages with Shallots and Kalamata Olives

Ingredients

1 lb sausages chopped

4 shallots, finely chopped

1/2 cup lemon juice (2 lemons)

16 black and green Kalamata olives

2 Tbsp whole grain mustard

4 Tbsp extra virgin olive oil

salt and ground black pepper to taste

Directions

1. Preheat oven to 400F. Grease an roasting pan and place in the sausages and chopped shallots.
2. Roast for 20 minutest.
3. When ready, remove the meat from the sausages and season with salt and freshly ground pepper to taste
4. Pour the lemon juice into the roasting tin.
5. Add in the mustard and chopped olives and simmer gently for 2-3 minutes. Pour lemon mixture over the sausages and shallots.
6. Place on serving plate and serve.

Servings: 6

Cooking Times

Total Time: 30 minutes

Nutrition Facts (per serving)

Total Carbohydrates: 14,9g

Dietary Fiber: 0,42g

Net Carbs: 6,78g

Protein: 18,48

Total Fat: 16,67g

Calories: 408

Spinach and Cheese Stuffed Mushrooms

Ingredients

12 large mushroom caps with stems

1 cream cheese

1 cup cooked, chopped spinach

1 Tbsp garlic, minced

1 tsp red pepper flakes

2 scallions, finely chopped

1 tsp salt

1 tsp fresh cracked pepper

3 tsp extra virgin olive oil

2 Tbsp almond, ground

2 Tbsp Parmesan cheese

1 tsp granulated garlic

1 Tbsp fresh flat leaf parsley, finely chopped

Directions

1. Preheat the oven to 400 degrees F.
2. First, remove the mushrooms stems. Chop the stems finely.
3. Heat a frying skillet with 2 teaspoons of olive oil and cook the mushrooms stems for 5 minutes.
4. In a bowl, combine the cream cheese, red pepper flakes, scallions, chopped spinach, minced garlic, cooked mushroom stems, salt and pepper.
5. In a small bowl, combine ground almonds, parmesan cheese, parsley and granulated garlic.
6. Fill the mushroom cavities with cheese and mushrooms mixture. Sprinkle the ground almonds mixture over each mushroom.

7. Drizzle the remaining 1 teaspoon of oil over the filling in the mushroom caps.
8. Bake in oven about 12 minutes.
9. Serve hot.

Servings: 6

Cooking Times

Preparation Time: 8 minutes

Cooking Time: 12 minutes

Total Time: 20 minutes

Nutrition Facts (per serving)

Total Carbohydrates: 11,36g

Dietary Fiber: 5,24g

Net Carbs: 6,98g

Protein: 11,75g

Total Fat: 6,36g

Calories: 138,32

Spinach-Chard Puree with Almonds

Ingredients

1 lb baby spinach leaves

1/2 lb Swiss chard, tough stems removed, tender stems and leaves torn into 2" pieces

1 cup cauliflower flowerets (1 cup)

1 leek

1/4 cup extra virgin olive oil

3 cups water

4 Tbsp toasted almond slivers

1/4 cup tofu cheese, cubed

salt and black ground pepper to taste

Directions

1. Wash the leek and cut it into thick slices.
2. Heat the olive oil in a saucepan and cook the leek and cauliflower for about 2-3 minutes.
3. Add the chard and cleaned spinach leaves, water and a pinch of salt and pepper to taste. Bring to the boil and let it simmer for 15 minutes.
4. Remove from the heat and place the vegetables in a food processor. Blend into a very smooth soup.
5. Pour the mixture into bowls, place some tofu cubes on top and generously sprinkle with ground toasted almonds.

Servings: 10

Cooking Times

Total Time: 35 minutes

Nutrition Facts (per serving)

Total Carbohydrates: 6,92g

Dietary Fiber: 1,88g

Net Carbs: 0,94g

Protein: 5,24g

Total Fat: 1,69g

Calories: 47,47

Lunch Recipes

Baked Creamy Cauliflower-Broccoli Chicken

Ingredients

2 boneless chicken breasts

1 cup chicken broth

3 cups cauliflower

3 cups broccoli, steamed and chopped

2 cups shredded Cheddar cheese

1 cup heavy cream

1 small yellow onion

1/2 Tbsp. minced garlic

1 tsp. lemon juice

1/2 cup mayonnaise

3 Tbsp. ghee

fresh parsley, chopped

salt and fresh pepper to taste

Directions

1. Preheat the oven to 350 degrees.
2. In a deep saucepot boil chicken breast until the chicken is cooked through.
3. Meanwhile, in a frying pan with the ghee cook up the garlic and onions on a low heat. Add all spices one by one stirring frequently.
4. While that's cooking, in a food processor blend up your cauliflower.
5. When the onions are soft, add the cauliflower. Cook for 2-3 minutes. Add in the chicken broth. Cook, covered for about 10 minutes.
6. Add the heavy cream and lemon juice and let simmer uncovered on low for about 10 minutes more. At the end, add in mayonnaise and stir.
7. Pull apart your chicken and add half of chicken into the cauliflower cream mixture.
8. Use the other half to line the bottom of an 8x8 casserole dish. On top of the chicken, layer in chopped broccoli.
9. Top with the cauliflower cream mixture.
10. Cover it with cheddar cheese.
11. Bake in preheated oven for 40 minutes. Serve hot.

Servings: 8

Cooking Times: 1 hour and 15 minutes

Nutrition Facts (per serving)

Calories 365, 49

Total Fat 29,17g 45%

Total Carbohydrates 9,25g 3%

Fiber 0,95g 4%

Protein 17,9g 36%

Baked Manchego Chicken Wings

Ingredients

20 frozen wings

1 cup of grated Manchego cheese (or Parmesan, Asagio...)

2 Tbsp. Olive oil

2 tsp. dried oregano

1/2 Tbsp. garlic powder

1 tsp. garlic salt

Directions

1. Preheat oven to 450F.
2. In a baking pan greased with olive oil place frozen chicken wings. Sprinkle with salt and oregano.
3. Bake for 35 minutes.
4. Remove from oven and toss in a bowl with another tbsp. of garlic oil until coated.
5. Sprinkle with grated Manchego cheese and garlic powder.
6. Serve hot.

Servings: 4

Cooking Times

Total Time: 45 minutes

Nutrition Facts (per serving)

Calories 446, 38

Total Fat 33,51g 52%

Total Carbohydrates 2,67g <1%

Fiber 0,68g 3%

Protein 32,34g 65%

Baked Pork Chops in Sweet-Sour Marinade

Ingredients

4.48 lbs. pork chops

1 cup Apple cider vinegar

1 cup Erythritol

4 Tbsp. soy Sauce

1 cup Apple Cider Vinegar

1 tsp. ginger

1 tsp. pepper

coconut or olive oil for greasing

Directions

1. Preheat oven to 350F.
2. In a food processor, add all of the ingredients (except the pork chops).
3. Blend well to make the marinade.
4. In a greased pan place all of the pork chops and pour the marinade over it.
5. Cook for 60 minutes in a preheated oven flipping after 30 minutes.
6. Once ready place chops on a serving plate and enjoy your lunch!

Servings: 10

Cooking Times

Preparation Time: 10 minutes

Total Time: 1 hour and 10 minutes

Nutrition Facts (per serving)

Calories 307, 86

Total Fat 6,97g 11%

Total Carbohydrates 11,43g 4%

Fiber 0,08g <1%

Protein 45,89g 92%

Bolognese Squash Spaghetti

Ingredients

1 lb. ground beef

2 1/2 cups Spaghetti squash

1 egg

3/4 cup Marinara Sauce

1 cup grated Parmesan cheese

1 cups shredded mozzarella cheese

1 tsp. chili powder

1/2 tsp. oregano

1/2 tsp. parsley (fresh and chopped)

1/2 tsp. basil

1 tsp. crushed red pepper flakes

2 tsp. of garlic minced

sea salt and ground fresh pepper to taste

ghee

Directions

1. Preheat oven to 350F.
2. Roast your spaghetti squash in the oven for about one hour.
3. In a saucepan, heat Marinara sauce; add oregano, parsley, basil and red pepper flakes. Cover and let simmer for a few minutes. Mix meatball ingredients in a bowl and roll into quarter-sized mini meatballs.

4. In a frying pan heat the ghee and cook meatballs covered. After 3 minutes, flip when halfway browned.
5. Once the meatballs are cooked through, transfer them into the sauce.
6. In a small bread pan, layer spaghetti squash, sauce, meatballs and mozzarella.
7. Bake on 25 for 30 minutes. Serve hot.

Servings: 5

Cooking Times

Total Time: 45 minutes

Nutrition Facts (per serving)

Calories 446, 8

Total Fat 30,63g 47%

Total Carbohydrates 9,1g 3%

Fiber 0,93g 4%

Protein 32,33g 65%

Cheesy Zoodles with Fresh Basil

Ingredients

2 cups zucchini noodles (zoodles)

2 Tbsp. fresh chopped basil

1/4 cup Pecorino Romano cheese, shaved

1/4 cup Grana Padano cheese, grated

3 Tbsp. salted butter

3 cloves mashed garlic

1 tsp. red pepper flakes

1 Tbsp. chopped red pepper

1 Tbsp. coconut oil

Salt and fresh cracked pepper to taste

Directions

1. In a frying pan over medium heat, melt butter and coconut oil. Add in garlic, chopped red pepper and red pepper flakes. Sauté for 1 minute only.

2. Add in the zoodles and let cook for 1-2 minutes. Turn off heat and toss with fresh basil. Toss slightly.

3. Add in Pecorino Romano cheese and toss.

4. Finally, sprinkle on top with grated Grana Padano cheese.

5. Serve immediately.

Servings: 3

Cooking Times

Total Time: 15 minutes

Nutrition Facts (per serving)

Calories 314, 18

Total Fat 26,38g 41%

Total Carbohydrates 6,18g 2%

Fiber 2,3g 9%

Protein 15,78g 32%

Spicy Spinach Casserole

Ingredients

2 1/2 cups spinach, drained

2 lbs. ground pork/beef

16 oz. cream cheese

10 Tbsp. sour cream

8 oz. Emmenthal Cheese, shredded

2 cups pepper sauce

1 onion

1 red pepper

4 tsp. Taco seasoning

Sliced Jalapeños to taste

Directions

1. Preheat oven to 350F. Grease one 8" square and a 9x13 baking dish.
2. Chop and sauté some jalapenos with chopped peppers and onions. Transfer to a bowl and set aside.
3. Add the spinach to the pan and cook until thawed completely. Move the spinach to the prep bowl
4. In a frying pan, add ground pork/meat and cook until browned well. Add taco seasoning and mix. Remove from fire and set aside.
5. In a bowl, add sour cream, mozzarella and cream cheese. Add in peppers, onion, spinach and ground meat.
6. Transfer this mix to prepared and greased baking dish and bake for 40 minutes.
7. Serve hot or cold.

Servings: 10

Cooking Times

Preparation Time: 15 minutes

Cooking Time: 45 minutes

Total Time: 1 hour

Nutrition Facts (per serving)

Calories 460, 42

Total Fat 37,26g 57%

Total Carbohydrates 5,33g 2%

Fiber 0,84g 3%

Protein 25,63g 51%

Cabbage with Ground Beef Stew

Ingredients

1 1/2 lb. ground beef

2 lbs. green cabbage

1/2 cup unsalted butter

1/2 cup water

3 cups pasta sauce

Salt and pepper to taste

Directions

1. In a food processor, shred quartered cabbage.
2. In a saucepan, melt the butter and add the cabbage, water and salt and pepper to taste.
3. Cover and cook for 12-15 minutes, stirring occasionally
4. In a meanwhile, in a frying pan brown the ground beefs.
5. Once browned, add the beef to the cabbage and stir well. Finally, add the pasta sauce and stir. Serve hot.

Servings: 10

Cooking Times

Cooking Time: 15 minutes

Total Time: 25 minutes

Nutrition Facts (per serving)

Calories 307, 99

Total Fat 22,29g 34%

Total Carbohydrates 12,34g 4%

Fiber 3,6g 14%

Protein 14,9g 30%

Three Cheeses & Beef Pizza

Ingredients

1 lb. ground beef

2 beef sausage

1 cup chopped Romaine lettuce

2 Tbsp. yellow onions

3 Tbsp. chopped dill pickle

1 1/2 cups Parmesan cheese

1/2 cup Colby cheese, shredded

1 1/2 cups Cheddar, shredded

1/4 Tbsp. paprika

1/4 tsp. Old Bay seasoning

1/4 tsp. garlic powder

1/4 tsp. onion powder

2 Tbsp. organic Thousand island dressing

mustard to taste

1/4 tsp. sea salt

1/4 tsp. ground black pepper

olive oil

2 Tbsp. water

Directions

1. In a frying pan greased with olive oil, add 1 cup Parmesan cheese evenly and then on top, 1 cup shredded Cheddar.
2. Leave to cook 2-3 minutes; use a spatula to lift the edges and underneath of the pizza, and slide out onto a flat surface. Allow to cool.
3. Repeat the same process, for the second pizza crust. Once done, set both cheese crusts aside.
4. Use a spatula and evenly spread Thousand Island dressing over the cheese crusts
5. In a frying pan add ground beef and cook until browned. Add old bay seasoning, garlic powder, onion powder paprika, 2 tbsp. water, salt, ground black pepper to taste. Mix and set to simmer on low.
6. Finally, add in chopped hot dogs into slices and simmer for about 4-5 minutes.
7. Place chopped lettuce over your pizza crust.
8. In a bowl, place your pickles, onions, Colby cheese, and set aside.
9. On top of each cheese crust, add about a cup of the ground meat and hotdog mixture and spread evenly .Sprinkle with onions and pickles.
10. Drizzle mustard on top.
11. Sprinkle with more cheese if you like and serve.

Servings: 7

Cooking Time: 20 minutes

Nutrition Facts (per serving)

Calories 511, 3

Total Fat 39,9g 61%

Total Carbohydrates 2,78g <1%

Fiber 0,42g 2%

Protein 33,59g 67%

Chicken Angel Eggs

Ingredients

1 cup chicken, finely chopped

6 eggs

3 Tbsp. mayonnaise

1 Tbsp. chopped onion

1/2 tsp. dill

1/2 tsp. parsley

1 tsp. Dijon mustard

1/2 tsp. pepper mix seasoning

old bay seasoning

salt and black ground pepper to taste

Directions

1. In a bowl, mix all rest of ingredients (except eggs) until well mixed. Refrigerate the chicken salad for 10-15 minutes.
2. Boil your eggs. Shell, cool, and cut in half. Save or toss your yolks.
3. Fill your egg halves with chicken salad. Sprinkle with Old Bay or some other seasoning of your taste. Serve.

Servings: 4

Cooking Times

Total Time: 25 minutes

Nutrition Facts (per serving)

Calories 161, 85

Total Fat 11,22g 17%

Total Carbohydrates 3,73g 1%

Fiber 0,08g <1%

Protein 10,82g 22%

Monterey Jack Steak

Ingredients

1 lb. shaved steak

4 slices Monterey Jack cheese

2 Tbsp. mayonnaise

1 Tbsp. Dijon mustard

1/4 cup chopped green peppers

1/4 cup chopped onions

1 Tbsp. minced garlic

1 Tbsp. olive oil

1 Tbsp. ghee

Directions

1. In a large frying pan add ghee and olive oil to warm over medium heat. Add onions, green peppers and garlic. Cook until soft, about 2-3 minutes. Add shaved steak and cook until browned several minutes.
2. Turn heat down to low. Add Dijon mustard and mayonnaise and mix.
3. Add Monterey Jack cheese on top of the steak and let melt until cheese is melted throughout, about 1 minute.
4. Serve hot.

Servings: 4

Cooking Times

Total Time: 20 minutes

Nutrition Facts (per serving)

Calories 345, 42

Total Fat 25,2g 39%

Total Carbohydrates 4,35g 1%

Fiber 0,48g 2%

Protein 24,51g 49%

Pumpkin Chili

Ingredients

2 lbs. ground beef

1 can (15 oz.) pumpkin puree

1 Tbsp. pumpkin pie spice

3 cups 100% tomato juice

3 tomatoes, diced

1 red bell pepper

1 yellow onion

2 tsp. cumin

1 Tbsp. chili powder

2 tsp. cayenne pepper

ghee or coconut oil

Directions

1. In a large frying pan greased with ghee or coconut oil, brown the meat over medium heat.

2. Chop the onion and pepper and add into the pot with the meat. Cook 3-5 minutes or until the onions become translucent.

3. Add in the rest of the ingredients and let simmer on LOW for 30 minutes.

4. Season chili with salt and pepper to taste and cook for another 30 minutes.

5.   Serve hot.

Servings: 8

Cooking Times

Total Time: 1 hour and 20 minutes

Nutrition Facts (per serving)

Calories 354, 83

Total Fat 25,24g 39%

Total Carbohydrates 9,87g 3%

Fiber 2,14g 9%

Protein 21,87g 44%

Slow Cooker Roast and Chicken Stew

Ingredients

3 lb. pot roast

1 lb. chicken breast (boiled and shredded)

6 oz. Italian sweet sausage

2 cups beef broth

1 cup chicken stock

1/2 medium onion (chopped)

1 can (11 oz.) low carb diced tomatoes

1/4 tsp. thyme

1/4 tsp. celery salt

1 Tbsp. coconut oil

1 tsp. basil

2 tsp. dried dill weed

2 tsp. garlic powder

2 tsp. pepper

1 Tbsp. garlic salt

1 tsp. minced garlic

1 Tbsp. oregano

1 Tbsp. powdered buttermilk

4 tsp. onion powder

4 tsp. dried parsley

5 tsp. red pepper flakes

2 tsp. hot sauce

Directions

1. At the bottom of your Slow Cooker place roast, chicken breast and Italian sausages. Add on the top all other ingredients and stir lightly.

2. Close the lid and cook on LOW for about 6-8 hours.

3. Once ready, flavor to taste with some additional hot sauce, salt and pepper to your own liking and serve hot.

Servings: 10

Nutrition Facts (per serving)

Calories 467, 06

Total Fat 36,21g 56%

Total Carbohydrates 3,76g 1%

Fiber 1,03g 4%

Protein 30,11g 60%

Mediterranean Pecorino Romano Breaded Cutlets

Ingredients

6 pork cutlets

1/2 cup grated Pecorino Romano cheese

2 Tbsp. fresh lemon juice

2 Tbsp. water

1 Tbsp. olive oil

1 Tbsp. green pepper, minced

1 Tbsp. garlic, minced

salt and ground black pepper to taste

Directions

1. Heat a greasing frying pan to medium.
2. In a bowl pour water, lemon juice, olive oil, minced pepper and garlic. Season the salt and pepper to taste. Mix well.
3. In a separate bowl pour grated Pecorino Romano cheese.
4. Dip each cutlet first in liquid dressing and then in cheese.
5. Cook cutlets in pan for about 15-20 minutes. Serve hot.

Servings: 3

Cooking Times

Total Time: 30 minutes

Nutrition Facts (per serving)

Calories 395, 93

Total Fat 38,78g 60%

Total Carbohydrates 2,5g <1%

Fiber 0,16g <1%

Protein 9,1g 18%

Oriental Garlicky Chicken Thighs

Ingredients

4 chicken thighs

16 whole cloves of garlic

2 Tbsp. ghee

2 Tbsp. juice of one fresh lemon

1 cup of baby carrots

1 onion, cut into quarters

2 tomatoes cut in half

3 Tbsp. garlic olive oil (or extra-virgin olive oil)

oregano

Salt and pepper

Directions

1. Preheat oven to 500F degrees.
2. Grease the bottom of a non-stick frying pan with garlic olive oil (or olive oil). Add in the chicken thighs together.
3. In between the thighs, wedge in the garlic gloves, onions, tomatoes and baby carrots.
4. Pour the lemon juice over the chicken thighs. Drizzle ghee and garlic oil over the thighs.
5. Sprinkle oregano over the dish and season with salt and pepper to taste.
6. Bake in preheated oven for 25-30 minutes.
7. Reduce heat to 350 and cook for 20 minutes more.
8. Once ready, let cool for 5 minutes on a wire rack and serve hot.

Servings: 4

Cooking Times

Total Time: 1 hour and 5 minutes

Nutrition Facts (per serving)

Calories 237, 52

Total Fat 14,52g 22%

Total Carbohydrates 8,97g 3%

Fiber 1,31g 5%

Protein 17,68g 35%

Pordenone Cauliflower Lasagna

Ingredients

12 chicken thighs

30 oz. chopped cauliflower

6 green onions

1 onion, chopped

1 green pepper

6 bacon Slices

1 cup Cream Cheese

1/2 cup heavy cream

8 oz. Pepper Jack Cheese, shredded

8 oz. Cheddar Cheese, shredded

1 Tbsp. garlic, minced

salt and pepper to taste

Directions

1. Preheat oven to350F.
2. Chop up a head of cauliflower into florets. Cook the cauliflower in the microwave on the vegetable setting. Set aside.
3. In a pan on stovetop, toss the chicken thighs with salt and pepper to taste. Add some water to about mid-thigh and cook for 60 minutes. Chop up the onions and peppers and pan fry it.
4. Add all of the other ingredients, reserving 2 oz. Cheddar and 2 oz. of Pepper Jack Cheese.

5. Add the mixture into a large, greased casserole dish and top with the remaining cheese.
6. Cover with foil and cook for 30 minutes. Serve hot.

Servings: 10

Cooking Times

Preparation Time: 20 minutes

Cooking Time: 1 hour and 30 minutes

Nutrition Facts (per serving)

Calories 486, 47

Total Fat 35,69g 55%

Total Carbohydrates 13,73g 5%

Fiber 2,2g 9%

Protein 28,09g 56%

Roasted Chicken & Prosciutto with Brussels sprouts

Ingredients

2 lbs. chicken tenderloins

4 oz. prosciutto

12 oz. Brussels sprouts

1/2 cup chicken broth

1 1/2 cups heavy cream

1 tsp. minced garlic

1 lemon, quartered and seeded

ghee or coconut oil for frying

Directions

1. Preheat oven to 400 degrees.
2. Cut the Brussels sprouts in half and boil for 5 minutes. Remove from heat and set aside.
3. In a frying pan add 1/2 cup chicken broth and bring to a boil on medium. After that, add heavy cream, minced garlic and lemon and let simmer for 5-10 minutes stirring frequently. Remove from heat and set aside.
4. In a separate frying pan, heat up some ghee and add chicken. Cook on medium high heat for several minutes, and then add chopped prosciutto until chicken is cooked.
5. In a small casserole dish (9×9) and layer from bottom to top: Brussels sprouts, chicken, prosciutto, lemon cream sauce on top.
6. Bake in preheated oven for 20 minutes. Serve hot.

Servings: 6

Cooking Times

Total Time: 40 minutes

Nutrition Facts (per serving)

Calories 333, 34

Total Fat 16,76g 26%

Total Carbohydrates 5,2g 2%

Fiber 1,48g 6%

Protein 39,47g 79%

Roquefort Spinach, Zoodles and Bacon Salad

Ingredients

4 cups of zucchini noodles

1 cup fresh broccoli

1/2 cup crumbled bacon

1 cup fresh spinach

1/3 cup Roquefort, bleu cheese, crumbled

1/3 cup bleu cheese dressing

fresh cracked pepper (to taste)

Directions

1. In a deep bowl add all the ingredients together and toss slightly with wooden spoon.
2. Serve and enjoy!

Servings: 5

Cooking Time: 5 minutes

Nutrition Facts (per serving)

Calories 81, 21

Total Fat 3,15g 5%

Total Carbohydrates 9,58g 3%

Fiber 3,05g 12%

Protein 6,07g 12%

Sour Avocado and Chicken Moussaka

Ingredients

8 chicken thighs, cooked

1 cup sour cream

1 cup Parmesan Cheese

4 avocados

1 onion

1 green pepper

1 Tbsp. cayenne peppers sauce

salt and ground pepper to taste

coconut oil for greasing

Directions

1. Preheat oven to 350 F. Grease a baking dish with coconut oil.
2. In a pot cook your chicken thighs about 35 minutes. Peel avocados, cut in half, and slice into thin strips.
3. Line the bottom with avocado slices. In a small pan fry chopped peppers and onions until caramelized.
4. Add the chicken into a large bowl and chop it. Add remaining ingredients and mix well.
5. Spoon mixture over the avocado slices. Bake for 20 minutes.
6. Serve hot.

Servings: 8

Cooking Times

Total Time: 35 minutes

Nutrition Facts (per serving)

Calories 345, 67

Total Fat 25,32g 39%

Total Carbohydrates 11,08g 4%

Fiber 6,45g 26%

Protein 20,98g 42%

Spicy Italian Sausage and Spinach Casserole

Ingredients

16 oz. spicy Italian sausage

2 1/2 cups frozen spinach

12 eggs

8 oz. Cheddar

1 onion

9 oz. Cherry Tomatoes

1 green pepper, chopped

12 Tbsp. Heavy Cream

Garlic powder

Onion Powder

Salt and ground pepper to taste

coconut or olive oil

Directions

1. Preheat oven to 350F. Grease casserole dish with coconut or olive oil.
2. In microwave cook the spinach. Chop the spicy Italian sausage and cook in a frying pan until browned. Remove to the big bowl and set aside.
3. In the same frying pan, cook the sliced onion and pepper. Transfer to the bowl with spinach.
4. Whisk together the eggs, spices and a heavy cream. Add the cheese to the bowl and combine, then add the egg mixture and combine.

5. Transfer to a greased casserole dish and add cherry tomatoes.
6. Cook in preheated oven for 50 minutes. Serve hot.

Servings: 10

Cooking Times

Total Time: 1 hour and 5 minutes

Nutrition Facts (per serving)

Calories 343, 5

Total Fat 25,91g 40%

Total Carbohydrates 6,27g 2%

Fiber 2,5g 10%

Protein 22,68g 45%

Squash Spaghetti Lasagna Dish

Ingredients

2 1/2 lbs. ground beef

2 large Spaghetti Squash

7 ounces whole milk Ricotta Cheese

7 ounces Mozzarella cheese, sliced

4 cups Marinara sauce

coconut or olive oil for greasing

Directions

1. Preheat oven to 375F. Grease a large baking dish with coconut or olive oil.
2. Split the Spaghetti Squash and lay face down into large glass dish and fill with water. Bake for 40-45 minutes.
3. While the Spaghetti Squash is cooking, in a large saucepan cook the ground meat and the marinara sauce. Once combined, set aside.
4. When the Spaghetti Squash is done scrap the meat of the squash to from spaghetti.
5. Assembly the lasagna in a large greased pan, start with a layer of Spaghetti Squash, then the meat sauce, then slices of mozzarella, then ricotta, then repeats until ingredients are exhausted.
6. Bake for 30-35 35 minutes until the top layer of cheese is browning. Serve hot or keep refrigerated.

Servings: 14

Cooking Times

Total Time: 1 hour and 30 minutes

Nutrition Facts (per serving)

Calories 437, 3

Total Fat 27,77g 43%

Total Carbohydrates 16,49g 5%

Fiber 1,91g 8%

Protein 28,79g 58%

Tuna Avocado Bites

Ingredients

Mayonnaise (1/4 cup)

Parmesan cheese (1/4 cup)

Garlic powder (1/2 teaspoon)

Salt

Canned Tuna (10 oz., drained)

Avocado (1, cubed)

Almond flour (1/3 cup)

Onion powder (1/4 teaspoon)

Coconut oil (1/2 cup)

Directions

1. Combine all ingredients in a bowl except oil and avocado.

2. Add avocado and fold, use hands to form balls and dust with flour.

3. Heat oil in a pot and fry tuna bites until golden all over.

4. Serve.

Servings: 12

Nutrition Facts (per serving)

Calories 135

Net Carbs 0.8g

Fats 11.8g

Protein 6.2 g

Fiber 1.2g

Note: 3-4 bites would be good for a serving. Paired with a salad and lunch is complete.

Crispy Baked Tofu and Bok Choy Salad

Ingredients

For Tofu:

Soy sauce (1 tablespoon)

Water (1 tablespoon)

Rice wine vinegar (1 tablespoon)

Tofu (15 oz., extra firm)

Sesame oil (1 tablespoon)

Garlic (2 teaspoons)

Lemon juice (from ½ lemon)

For Salad:

Green onion (1 stalk)

Coconut oil (3 tablespoons)

Sambal Olek (1 tablespoon)

Lime juice (from ½ lime)

Bok Choy (9 oz.)

Cilantro (2 tablespoons, chopped)

Soy sauce (2 tablespoons)

Peanut butter (1 tablespoon)

Stevia liquid (7 drops)

Directions

1. Wrap tofu in a clean cloth and press for 6 hours until dry.

2. Combine soy sauce, water, vinegar, lemon juice, sesame oil and garlic in a bowl and cube tofu. Add to marinade, cover with plastic and put aside for 30 minutes or overnight if possible.

3. Set oven to 350 °F. Use parchment paper to line a baking sheet and place marinated tofu on sheet. Bake for 35 minutes.

4. Prepare dressing for salad by combining all ingredients except bok choy. Chop bok choy finely and toss in dressing.

5. Top bok choy with baked tofu and serve.

Servings: 3

Nutrition Facts (per serving)

Calories 442

Net Carbs 5.7g

Fats 35g

Protein 25 g

Fiber 1.7g

Homemade Meatballs

Ingredients

500g ground beef

1 whole egg

Almond flour (1/2 cups)

2 cloves of garlic, minced

Oregano, dried (1 teaspoon)

Thyme, dried (1 teaspoon)

1 cup mozzarella cheese, shredded

Salt and pepper to taste

Homemade marinara sauce (1/2 cups)

Directions

1. Preheat oven at 450F.

2. In a large bowl, place the ground beef, egg, almond flour, garlic, oregano, thyme, and season with salt and pepper. Also add the cheese.

3. Using your hands, mix all the ingredients together; making sure that everything is well combined.

4. Create 25 pcs of meat balls and lay them on a baking sheet lined with parchment paper.

5. Cook in the oven to cook for 15 minutes or until golden brown.

6. Serve the meatballs with marinara sauce.

Servings: 12

Nutrition Facts (per serving)

Calories: 117

Net Carbs: 0.9

Fat: 9.3g

Protein: 7g

BBQ Chicken Soup

Ingredients

For Soup Base:

Chicken thighs (3)

Salt

Chicken broth (1 ½ cups)

Chili seasoning (2 teaspoons)

Olive oil (2 tablespoons)

Beef broth (1 ½ cups)

Black pepper

For BBQ Sauce:

Ketchup (1/4 cup, reduced sugar)

Dijon mustard (2 tablespoons)

Hot sauce (1 tablespoon)

Worcestershire sauce (1 teaspoon)

Onion powder (1 teaspoon)

Red chili flakes (1 teaspoon)

Butter (1/4 cup)

Tomato paste (1/4 cup)

Soy sauce (1 tablespoon)

Liquid smoke (2 ½ teaspoons)

Garlic powder (1 ½ teaspoons)

Chili powder (1 teaspoon)

Cumin (1 teaspoon)

Directions

1. Set oven to 400 ℉. Remove bones from chicken and put bones aside. Season chicken with chili seasoning and place into oven for 50 minutes.
2. Heat oil in a deep pot and add bones. Cook for 5 minutes then add beef and chicken broth; season with pepper and salt.
3. Take chicken from oven and remove skin. Add the fat to the soup and mix together. Combine BBQ sauce ingredients and add to pot. Cook for 30 minutes.
4. Combine fats in soup by using an immersion blender then shred chicken and add to soup. Cook for 20 minutes.
5. Serve topped with chicken skin. May add cheese or bell peppers.

Servings: 4

Nutrition Facts (per serving)

Calories 487

Net Carbs 4.3g

Fats 38.3g

Protein 24.5 g

Fiber 1.3g

Salmon Salad in Avo Cups

Ingredients

1 medium-sized salmon fillet

1 pc. shallot, diced

Mayo (1/4 cups)

½ juice of lime

Fresh dill, chopped (2 tablespoons)

Ghee (1 tablespoon)

1 large avocado, sliced in half and pitted

salt and pepper to taste

Directions

1. Preheat oven at 400F

2. Place the salmon fillet on a baking sheet and drizzle it with ghee and juice of lime. Season with salt and pepper and place in the oven to cook for 20-25 minutes.

3. When done, allow the salmon to cook for a few minutes and shred using a fork.

4. Place the salmon in a bowl, add the diced shallot, and mix well.

5. Add the dill and mayo to the salmon mixture and combine well. Set aside.

6. Remove the insides of the avocado halves making sure that the skin is still intact to make cups.

7. Mash the avocado meat in a bowl and then add to the salmon mixture. Combine well.

8. Transfer the avocado and salmon salad back to the avocado cups and serve.

Servings: 2

Nutrition Facts (per serving)

Calories: 463

Net Carbs: 6.4g

Fat: 35g

Protein: 27g

Bacon Chicken Patties

Ingredients

Chicken breast (12 oz. can)

Bell peppers (2, medium)

Parmesan cheese (1/4 cup)

Coconut flour (3 tablespoons)

Bacon (4 slices)

Sundried Tomato pesto (1/4 cup)

Egg (1)

Directions

1. Cook bacon until crisp, put aside until needed.

2. Put bell pepper into a processor and pulse until fine, put into a bowl and squeeze out excess liquid.

3. Put bacon and chicken into processor and pulse until thoroughly combined, transfer mixture to bowl with peppers.

4. Add egg, pesto parmesan and flour to mixture and combine.

5. Heat oil in a skillet and form patties. Add to pan and cook until golden all over.

6. Serve.

Servings: 10

Nutrition Facts (per serving)

Calories 159

Net Carbs 1.7g

Fats 11.5g

Protein 9.9 g

Fiber 14g

Savory Mince

Ingredients

Coconut oil (4 tablespoons)

1Kg Beef/Chicken/Lamb/Pork/Ostrich mince

2 Onion finely diced

Vegetables (green/red/yellow/orange peppers, mushroom, tomatoes, celery, baby marrows, spinach) finely diced (4 cups)

4 Carrots finely grated

1 Packet gluten free gravy

Tomato paste (1/2 cups)

250ml chicken stock

Directions

1. Heat coconut oil in a pan and fry chopped onion,

2. Add beef mince with and tomato paste and fry.

3. Add chopped vegetables and grated carrot to the cooked mince.

4. Continue to cook on a low heat until the vegetables are well cooked.

5. If your mixture seems to be drying out, keep adding chicken stock to keep at the right consistency.

6. The longer you cook this mixture, the more the flavours will infuse through the mince.

7. Add gluten free gravy.

Cheesy Bacon Spinach Log

Ingredients

Cheddar cheese (2 ½ cups, shredded)

Chipotle seasoning (2 tablespoons)

Bacon (30 slices)

Mrs. Dash seasoning (2 teaspoons)

Spinach (5 cups)

Directions

1. Set oven to 375 ℉.
2. Place bacon in a weaving pattern on a baking sheet lined with foil and season with spices.
3. Top bacon with cheese leaving a 1 inch space all around the edge. Add spinach and push it down and roll the bacon together into a log.
4. Sprinkle with salt and place into oven for 60 minutes.
5. Cool for 15 minutes and slice.
6. Serve.

Servings: 5

Nutrition Facts (per serving)

Calories 432

Net Carbs 3g

Fats 38.2g

Protein 32.8 g

Fiber 3g

Beef Sausage, Bacon & Broccoli Casserole

Ingredients

500 g beef sausage

1/2 head of broccoli

8 slices of bacon

Cream (1/2 cups)

Dijon mustard (1 tablespoon)

100 g grated cheddar cheese

Directions

1. Preheat oven to 350F
2. Slice the sausage and place in a small baking dish.
3. Slice the bacon and add to the sausage.
4. Break the broccoli into florets and arrange between the meat.
5. Mix the cream and mustard in a bowl and pour it all over the casserole, then top with the cheese.
6. Bake in the oven for 35 minutes.

Servings: 2

Nutrition Facts (per serving)

Calories: 300

Net Carbs: 3g

Fat: 25g

Protein: 20g

Grilled Cheese and Ham Sandwich

Ingredients

For buns:

Eggs (2)

Salted butter (1 ½ tablespoons)

Coconut flour (1 teaspoon)

Almond flour (3/4 cup)

Coconut oil (2 tablespoons)

Baking powder (1 teaspoon)

Salt (1/4 teaspoon)

Filling:

Deli Ham (4 slices)

Cheddar cheese (2 slices)

Butter (1 tablespoon, salted)

Muenster cheese (2 slices)

Directions

1. Set oven to 350 °F.

2. Place almond flour, baking powder in a bowl and mix together.

3. Put coconut oil and butter in a microwavable dish and heat until melted then add to dry mix. Combine until mixture gets doughy.

4. Beat eggs and add to dough mixture then put in coconut flour.

5. Grease cupcake molds and add batter to each about ¾ ways filled. Baked for 18 minutes and take from oven, allow to cool and slice into two horizontally.

6. Use cheese and ham to fill buns, melt butter in a skillet and place sandwiches into pan. Cook for 3 minutes on each side until golden and cheese melts.

7. Serve.

Servings: 1

Nutrition Facts (per serving)

Calories 272

Net Carbs 1.8g

Fats 24.2g

Protein 11.3g

Fiber 3.8g

Creamed Spinach

Ingredients

Spinach (2 cups)

½ small onion, chopped

Water (1/4 cups)

1/2 stock cube

1 clove of garlic, chopped

Heavy cream (1/4 cups)

Butter (2 tablespoons)

Salt and pepper to taste

Directions

1. Place spinach and onion to a pan with water and heat over medium-high fire.

2. Add stock cube and garlic and allow to steam for 8-10 minutes or until all the water has evaporated and the spinach is very soft.

3. Pour in the heavy cream and butter and then season with salt and pepper. Cooking until it thickens.

4. Using a hand-held blender blitz the spinach until fairly smooth.

5. Serve while hot

Servings: 1

Nutrition Facts (per serving)

Calories: 200

Net Carbs: 3g

Fat: 23g

Protein: 7g

Cheesy Pizza

Ingredients

Ground beef (1/2 lb.)

Eggs (2)

Garlic powder (1 teaspoon)

Basil (1/4 teaspoon)

Turmeric (1/4 teaspoon)

Cream cheese (8 oz., room temp.)

Chorizo sausage (1)

Parmesan cheese (1/4 cup, grated)

Cumin (1/2 teaspoon)

Italian seasoning (1/2 teaspoon)

Tomato sauce (3/4 cup, low carb)

Salt

Black pepper

Directions

1. Set oven to 375 F.

2. Put cream cheese, eggs, garlic powder, parmesan cheese and black pepper in a bowl and use mixer to blend until smooth.

3. Grease a baking pan and pour in cheese mixture and spread evenly; bake for 15 minutes.

4. Put beef into a skillet and cook for 5 minutes then add Italian seasoning, basil, salt, black pepper, cumin and turmeric. Cook for 10 minutes or until thoroughly cooked.

5. Take crust from oven and cool for 10 minutes then top with tomato sauce and cheese. Return to oven and bake for 10 minutes until cheese melts then top with beef.

6. Broil for an additional 5 minutes. Take from oven and cool for 10 minutes.

7. Slice and serve.

Servings: 12 small slices

Nutrition Facts (per serving)

Calories 145

Net Carbs 1.2g

Fats 11.3g

Protein 8.2 g

Fiber 3g

Hearty Portobello Burgers

Ingredients

Coconut oil (1/2 tablespoon)

Oregano (1 teaspoon)

Portobello mushroom caps (2)

Garlic (1 clove)

Salt

Black pepper

Dijon mustard (1 tablespoon)

Cheddar cheese (1/4 cup)

Beef/bison (6 oz.)

Directions

1. Heat griddle and combine spices and oil in a bowl.

2. Remove gills from mushrooms and place into marinade until needed.

3. Add beef, cheese, salt, mustard and pepper in another bowl and mix to combine; form into a patty.

4. Place marinated caps onto grill and cook for 8 minutes until thoroughly heated. Place patty onto grill and cook on each side for 5 minutes.

5. Take 'buns' from grill and top with burger and any other toppings you choose.

6. Serve.

Servings: 1

Nutrition Facts (per serving)

Calories 735

Net Carbs 4g

Fats 48g

Protein 60g

Fiber 4g

Chicken and Broccoli filled Zucchini

Ingredients

Butter (2 tablespoons)

Broccoli (1 cup)

Sour cream (2 tablespoons)

Zucchini (10 oz.)-2

Cheddar cheese (3 oz., shredded)

Rotisserie chicken (6 oz., shredded)

Green onion (1 stalk)

Salt

Black pepper

Directions

1. Set oven to 400 °F.

2. Slice zucchinis in half lengthwise and use spoons to remove cores. Melt butter and pour equally into each zucchini shell. Add black pepper and salt and bake for 20 minutes.

3. Chop broccoli and place into a bowl with sour cream and chicken. Fill zucchini boats with chicken mixture and top with cheese.

4. Bake for 15 minutes more or until golden.

5. Serve topped with green onion.

Servings: 2

Nutrition Facts (per serving)

Calories 476.5

Net Carbs 5g

Fats 34g

Protein 30 g

Fiber 3g

Super-Fast Egg Drop Soup

Ingredients

Chicken broth (1 ½ cups)

Butter (1 tablespoon)

Chili garlic paste (1 teaspoon)

Chicken bouillon (1/2 cube)

Eggs (2)

Directions

1. Add butter to pan, heat until it melts then add broth and bouillon
2. Bring to a boil and add chili paste, stir to combine and remove from flame.
3. Beat eggs in a bowl and add to broth, stir and put aside for a few minutes.
4. Serve.

Servings: 2

Nutrition Facts (per serving)

Calories 279

Net Carbs 2.5g

Fats 23g

Protein 12g

Fiber 0g

Salmon Salad in Avocado Cups

Ingredients

1 medium-sized salmon fillet

1 pc. Shallot, diced

¼ cup mayo

½ juice of lime

2 tsps. Fresh dill, chopped

1 tbsp. ghee

1 large avocado, sliced in half and pitted

salt and pepper to taste

Directions

1. Preheat oven at 400F
2. Place the salmon fillet on a baking sheet and drizzle it with ghee and juice of lime. Season with salt and pepper and place in the oven to cook for 20-25 minutes.
3. When done, allow the salmon to cook for a few minutes and shred using a fork.
4. Place the salmon in a bowl, add the diced shallot, and mix well.
5. Add the dill and mayo to the salmon mixture and combine well. Set aside.
6. Remove the insides of the avocado halves making sure that the skin is still intact to make cups.
7. Mash the avocado meat in a bowl and then add to the salmon mixture. Combine well.
8. Transfer the avocado and tuna salad back to the avocado cups and serve.

Servings: 2

Nutrition Facts (per serving)

Calories: 463

Net Carbs: 6.4g

Fat: 35g

Protein: 27g

Cheesy Hotdog Pockets

Ingredients

2 pcs. beef hot dogs

2 thick sticks of quick-melt cheese (or mozzarella)

4 slices of bacon

1/8 tsp. garlic powder

1/8 tsp. onion powder

salt and pepper to taste

Directions

1. Preheat oven at 400F
2. Cut the hotdogs lengthwise to create slits.
3. Insert the cheese sticks in the hotdog and then wrap the bacon with to the beef hotdog. Secure the bacon using a toothpick.
4. Transfer the hotdogs on a baking sheet lined with foil and flavor with garlic and onion powder.
5. Place in the oven to cook for 40 minutes or until the hotdogs turns golden brown and the cheese is melted,
6. Serve with a veggie salad on the side.

Nutritional Info (per serving)

Calories: 378

Net Carbs: 0.3 g

Fat: 35g

Protein: 17g

Beef Shred Salad

Ingredients

2 cups beef, shredded

1 yellow pepper, sliced thin lengthwise

1 white onion, sliced lengthwise

6 pcs. butter lettuce

2 tsp. mayo

1/8 tsp. chili flakes

Directions

1. Place the butter lettuces on a serving plate. Spread mayo on the lettuce and top with the shredded beef.
2. Place pepper slices and onions on top and season with chili flakes.
3. Serve as it is or rolled.

Nutritional Info (per serving)

Calories: 338

Net Carbs: 2.4

Fat: 25g

Protein: 24g

Spicy Chicken Thighs

Ingredients

2 lb. chicken thighs

¼ cup ghee or olive oil

½ tsp. garlic powder

½ tsp. paprika

½ tsp. cumin, ground

¼ tsp. cayenne

¼ tsp. coriander, ground

1/8 tsp. cinnamon, ground

1/8 tsp. ginger powder

1 tsp. salt

1 tsp. yellow curry

Directions

1. Preheat oven at 425F.
2. In a small bowl mix all the spices to create a dry rub.
3. Pat dry the chicken using a kitchen paper towel and place on a baking sheet lined with greased parchment paper.
4. Generously brush the chicken with ghee or olive oil.
5. Rub the spices to the chicken thighs making sure that you cover every side.
6. Place the chicken in the oven to cook for 50 minutes.
7. Let it cool before serving.

Nutritional Info (per serving)

Calories: 227

Net Carbs: .6g

Fat: 20g

Protein: 21g

Spring Roll in a Bowl

Ingredients

500g pork mince

2 cups cabbage, shredded finely

2 cup grated carrot

2 cups grated baby marrows

1 cup mushrooms

4 tbsp. coconut Oil

1/2 cup soya sauce

1 cup chicken stock

2 tsp. vinegar

5 cloves garlic, minced

4 tsp. grated ginger

4 finely sliced spring onions

½ cup toasted sesame seeds

1 hard-boiled egg, chopped

Directions

1. Heat the coconut oil and fry the garlic, spring onions, ginger.
2. Add the pork mince and brown.
3. Add the cabbage and carrot to the pot and toss to combine. Stir in the soy sauce.
4. Cover and cook until the vegetables are soft, about 15 minutes.
5. Dish up; add chopped hard-boiled egg over each of the bowls.
6. Garnish with sesame seeds once you have dished up.

Nutritional Info (per serving)

Calories: 80

Net Carbs: 5g

Fat: 5g

Protein: 3g

Green Salad

(This salad is the salad that is referred to across other meals)

Ingredients

1 cup green beans, steamed lightly

1 cup broccoli florets, steamed lightly

1 small tomato, finely sliced

1 cup lettuce

1 round feta

¼ cup toasted sunflower seeds, roasted

1 hard-boiled egg, chopped

For dressing:

1 tbsp. olive oil

Salt and pepper to taste

juice from ½ lemon

Directions

1. Place all the vegetables in a salad bowl.
2. Crumble the feta and sprinkle it along with the roasted pumpkin seeds and egg on top of the salad.
3. In a small bowl, pour the olive oil, add lemon juice, then add salt and pepper, and whisk together. Drizzle this dressing on top of the salad.
4. Toss gently before serving.

Nutritional Info (per serving)

Calories: 45

Net Carbs: 3g

Fat: 3g

Protein: 1g

Greek Salad

Ingredients

50g Grilled Chicken Breast

2 cups lettuce

10 Olives

½ Round Feta

5 Cherry Tomatoes

¼ Cucumber

1Tblsp Olive Oil

1tsp Lemon juice

Directions

1. Place all ingredients into a bowl, mix and enjoy!

Bacon, Lettuce, Tomato Salad

Ingredients

1 cup of lettuce

1 spring onion

1 tomato

¼ cup toasted pumpkin seeds

grated boiled egg

sliced avocado

4 rashes of crispy bacon (crumbled)

For dressing:

1 Tbsp. apple cider vinegar

1 tsp. lemon juice

½ a finely crushed clove of garlic

1 Tbsp. Olive oil and some finely crushed fresh ginger (optional)

Directions

1. In a large bowl combine salad ingredients
2. This can all be done at home and taken to work.

For dressing:

1. In a separate container mix dressing ingredients
2. Allow the dressing to sit for a few hours.

Pour the dressing over the salad when you are ready to eat.

Broccoli Salad

Ingredients

1 cup broccoli

2 medium celery stalks

1/2 cup mushroom pieces (fried)

1/4 cup Cherry tomatoes

1Tblsp olive oil

2 cups Lettuce

1Tblsp Balsamic Vinegar

125ml pumpkin seeds roasted dry in a pan.

Directions

1. Place all ingredients into a bowl, mix and enjoy!

Tuna/Smoked Salmon Salad

Ingredients

1 Tin Tuna in Water/100g Smoked Salmon

1 Hard Boiled Egg

½ Avo

1 Cup Green Beans (Steamed)

5 Cherry Tomatoes

1 Tbsp. Red Onion

½ Cup Celery

Directions

1. Place all ingredients into a bowl, mix and enjoy!

Avo & Tuna Lettuce Wraps

In a medium bowl, combine all ingredients for tuna salad. Mix with a fork. Refrigerate. To assemble, spoon tuna mixture into lettuce leaves. Top with avocado and tomato.

Warm Chicken Salad

Ingredients

1. Roast 2 medium chicken thighs in the oven the night before and remove meat from bones (eat skin whilst warm).

2. Reheat Chicken the following day and add to salad

Hearty Salad

Ingredients

1 Hard Boiled Egg grated

2 slices of country ham, finely sliced

30g cheddar cheese

1 tomato finely diced

2Tblsp Mayo

1 cup finely sliced crispy lettuce

2 spring onions finely chopped

½ green pepper finely chopped

Directions

1. Combine all the ingredients and then add the mayo and mix.

Crunchy Chicken Waldorf Salad

Ingredients

150ml full cream plain yogurt

1Tblsp Mayonnaise

2 teaspoons lemon juice

1/4 teaspoon salt

50g chopped cooked chicken breast

½ medium green apple, finely diced

1 cup finely sliced celery

1/2 cup chopped walnuts, toasted.

Directions

1. Whisk mayonnaise, yogurt, lemon juice and salt in a large bowl.
2. Add chicken, apple, celery and 1/4 cup walnuts.
3. Stir to coat well.
4. Serve topped with the remaining 1/4 cup walnuts.

Spinach Cheese & Bacon Log

Ingredients

Cheddar cheese (2 ½ cups, shredded)

Chipotle seasoning (2 tablespoons)

Bacon (30 slices)

Mrs. Dash seasoning (2 teaspoons)

Spinach (5 cups)

Directions

1. Set oven to 375 ℉.
2. Place bacon in a weaving pattern on a baking sheet lined with foil and season with spices.
3. Top bacon with cheese leaving a 1 inch space all around the edge. Add spinach and push it down and roll the bacon together into a log.
4. Sprinkle with salt and place into oven for 60 minutes.
5. Cool for 15 minutes and slice.
6. Serve.

Servings: 5

Nutrition Facts (per serving)

Calories 432

Net Carbs 3g

Fats 38.2g

Protein 32.8 g

Fiber 3g

Beef Sausage, Bacon & Broccoli Casserole

Ingredients

500 g beef sausage

1/2 head of broccoli

8 slices of bacon

Cream (1/2 cups)

Dijon mustard (1 tablespoon)

100 g grated cheddar cheese

Directions

1. Preheat oven to 350F
2. Slice the sausage and place in a small baking dish.
3. Slice the bacon and add to the sausage.
4. Break the broccoli into florets and arrange between the meat.
5. Mix the cream and mustard in a bowl and pour it all over the casserole, then top with the cheese.
6. Bake in the oven for 35 minutes.

Nutritional Information

Calories: 300

Net Carbs: 3g

Fat: 25g

Protein: 20g

Zucchini Stuffed with Chicken & Broccoli

Ingredients

Butter (2 tablespoons)

Broccoli (1 cup)

Sour cream (2 tablespoons)

Zucchini (10 oz.)-2

Cheddar cheese (3 oz., shredded)

Rotisserie chicken (6 oz., shredded)

Green onion (1 stalk)

Salt

Black pepper

Directions

1. Set oven to 400°F.
2. Slice zucchinis in half lengthwise and use spoons to remove cores. Melt butter and pour equally into each zucchini shell. Add black pepper and salt and bake for 20 minutes.
3. Chop broccoli and place into a bowl with sour cream and chicken. Fill zucchini boats with chicken mixture and top with cheese.
4. Bake for 15 minutes more or until golden.
5. Serve topped with green onion.

Servings: 2

Nutrition Facts (per serving)

Calories 476.5

Net Carbs 5g

Fats 34g

Protein 30 g

Fiber 3g

Beef Pumpkin Chili

Ingredients

2 lbs. ground beef

1 can (15 oz.) pumpkin puree

1 Tbsp. pumpkin pie spice

3 cups 100% tomato juice

3 tomatoes, diced

1 red bell pepper

1 yellow onion

2 tsp. cumin

1 Tbsp. chili powder

2 tsp. cayenne pepper

ghee or coconut oil

Directions

1. In a large frying pan greased with ghee or coconut oil, brown the meat over medium heat.
2. Chop the onion and pepper and add into the pot with the meat. Cook 3-5 minutes or until the onions become translucent.
3. Add in the rest of the ingredients and let simmer on LOW for 30 minutes.
4. Season chili with salt and pepper to taste and cook for another 30 minutes.
5. Serve hot.

Servings: 8

Cooking Time: 1 hour and 20 minutes

Nutrition Facts (per serving)

Total Carbs 9,87g

Calories 354, 83

Total Fat 25,24g

Fiber 2,14g

Sugar 5,5g

Protein 21,87g

Slow Cooker Chicken Stew

Ingredients

3 lb. pot roast

1 lb. chicken breast (boiled and shredded)

6 oz. Italian sweet sausage

2 cups beef broth

1 cup chicken stock

1/2 medium onion (chopped)

1 can (11 oz.) low carb diced tomatoes

1/4 tsp. thyme

1/4 tsp. celery salt

1 Tbsp. coconut oil

1 tsp. basil

2 tsp. dried dill weed

2 tsp. garlic powder

2 tsp. pepper

1 Tbsp. garlic salt

1 tsp. minced garlic

1 Tbsp. oregano

1 Tbsp. powdered buttermilk

4 tsp. onion powder

4 tsp. dried parsley

5 tsp. red pepper flakes

2 tsp. hot sauce

Directions

1. At the bottom of your Slow Cooker place roast, chicken breast and Italian sausages. Add on the top all other ingredients and stir lightly.
2. Close the lid and cook on LOW for about 6-8 hours.
3. Once ready, flavor to taste with some additional hot sauce, salt and pepper to your own liking and serve hot.

Servings: 8

Nutrition Facts (per serving)

Total Carbs 3,76g 1%

Calories 467, 06

Total Fat 36,21g 56%

Fiber 1,03g 4%

Sugar 0,59g

Protein 30,11g 60%

Pecorino Romano Breaded Cutlets

Ingredients

6 pork cutlets

1/2 cup grated Pecorino Romano cheese

2 Tbsp. fresh lemon juice

2 Tbsp. water

1 Tbsp. olive oil

1 Tbsp. green pepper, minced

1 Tbsp. garlic, minced

salt and ground black pepper to taste

Directions

1. Heat a greasing frying pan to medium.
2. In a bowl pour water, lemon juice, olive oil, minced pepper and garlic. Season the salt and pepper to taste. Mix well.
3. In a separate bowl pour grated Pecorino Romano cheese.
4. Dip each cutlet first in liquid dressing and then in cheese.
5. Cook cutlets in pan for about 15-20 minutes. Serve hot.

Servings: 3

Cooking Time: 30 minutes

Nutrition Facts (per serving)

Total Carbs 2,5g

Calories 395, 93

Total Fat 38,78g

Fiber 0,16g

Sugar 0,37g

Protein 9,1g

Garlic Chicken Thighs

Ingredients

4 chicken thighs

16 whole cloves of garlic

2 Tbsp. ghee

2 Tbsp. juice of one fresh lemon

1 cup of baby carrots

1 onion, cut into quarters

2 tomatoes cut in half

3 Tbsp. garlic olive oil (or extra-virgin olive oil)

oregano

Salt and pepper

Directions

1. Preheat oven to 500F degrees.
2. Grease the bottom of a non-stick frying pan with garlic olive oil (or olive oil). Add in the chicken thighs together.
3. In between the thighs, wedge in the garlic gloves, onions, tomatoes and baby carrots.
4. Pour the lemon juice over the chicken thighs. Drizzle the ghee and garlic oil over the thighs.
5. Sprinkle oregano over the dish and season with salt and pepper to taste.
6. Bake in preheated oven for 25-30 minutes.
7. Reduce heat to 350 and cook for 20 minutes more.
8. Once ready, let cool for 5 minutes on a wire rack and serve hot.

Servings: 4

Cooking Time: 1 hour and 5 minutes

Nutrition Facts (per serving)

Total Carbs 8,97g

Calories 237, 52

Total Fat 14,52g

Fiber 1,31g

Sugar 2,67g

Protein 17,68g

Chicken & Cauliflower Lasagna

Ingredients

12 chicken thighs

30 oz. chopped cauliflower

6 green onions

1 onion, chopped

1 green pepper

6 bacon Slices

1 cup Cream Cheese

1/2 cup heavy cream

8 oz. Pepper Jack Cheese, shredded

8 oz. Cheddar Cheese, shredded

1 Tbsp. garlic, minced

salt and pepper to taste

Directions

1. Preheat oven to350F.
2. Chop up a head of cauliflower into florets. Cook the cauliflower in the microwave on the vegetable setting. Set aside.
3. In a pan on stovetop, toss the chicken thighs with salt and pepper to taste. Add some water to about mid-thigh and cook for 60 minutes. Chop up the onions and peppers and pan fry it.
4. Add all of the other ingredients, reserving 2 oz. Cheddar and 2 oz. of Pepper Jack Cheese.
5. Add the mixture into a large, greased casserole dish and top with the remaining cheese.
6. Cover with foil and cook for 30 minutes. Serve hot.

Servings: 10

Preparation Time: 20 minutes

Cooking Time: 1 hour and 30 minutes

Nutrition Facts (per serving)

Total Carbs 13,73g

Calories 486, 47

Total Fat 35,69g

Fiber 2,2g

Sugar 2,93g

Protein 28,09g

Dinner Recipes

Baked Cheesy Meatballs

Ingredients

1 lb. ground beef (lean)

2 white onion

1 cup grated Cheddar cheese

4 oz. Gruyere cheese

1 egg

1.5 tsp. nutmeg

1.5 tsp. allspice

sea salt and freshly black pepper to taste

butter for greasing

Directions

1. Preheat oven to 350F.
2. In a greased frying pan, sauté onions until translucent. Remove from heat, and let cool.
3. In a food processor mince the Gruyere cheese. Set aside.
4. In a mixing bowl, whisk egg with grated Cheddar cheese. Add the spices, salt, and pepper and mix.
5. Add in onions and Gruyere cheese. Mix well until smooth.
6. Add the beef and mix until all ingredients are combined well.
7. Divide meat mixture and roll each piece into a ball.
8. Place the meatballs on a cookie sheet, and bake in preheated oven about 20 minutes. Serve hot.

Servings: 6

Cooking Times

Total Time: 35 minutes

Nutrition Facts (per serving)

Calories 385, 89

Total Fat 29,05g

Total Carbohydrates 4,79g

Fiber 0,91g

 Protein 25,25g

Chicken & Endive Casserole

Ingredients

1 endive head, cut into wide strips

1 1/2 lbs. skinless boneless chicken thighs

1 Tbsp. dried oregano

2 cups chopped onions

4 celery stalks, chopped

4 garlic cloves, chopped

1 cup diced tomatoes in juice

2 Tbsp. olive oil

8 cups water

Directions

1. In a large saucepan heat oil over medium-high heat.

2. Sprinkle the chicken with salt, pepper, and oregano. Add chicken in a saucepan. Mix in onions, celery and garlic. Sauté until vegetables begin to soften, about 4-5minutes.

3. Stir in tomatoes. Add broth; bring to boil. Reduce heat to medium; simmer until vegetables and chicken are tender, about 15 minutes.

4. Add endive hearts; simmer until wilted, about 3 minutes. Season with salt and pepper.

5. Ladle into bowls and serve hot.

Servings: 6

Cooking Times

Total Time: 40 minutes

Nutrition Facts (per serving)

Calories 144, 48

Total Fat 7,21g 11%

Total Carbohydrates 9,94g 3%

Fiber 2,05g 8%

Protein 9,89g 20%

Creamy Smoked Turkey Salad with Almonds

Ingredients

Salad ingredients

2 cups diced, cooked smoked turkey breast

1/4 cup sliced almonds

1/2 cup diced celery

1/4 cup sliced green onions

1/4 cup shredded cabbage

Dressing ingredients

4 oz. mayonnaise

2 oz. sour cream

2 drops sweet liquid Splenda

1 tsp. curry powder

Salt and pepper to taste

Directions

1. In a bowl, combine sour cream and mayonnaise and whisk until smooth. Add the spices and continue to whisk until smooth.
2. In a big bowl, combine all salad ingredients and the dressing and toss well. Serve and enjoy!

Note: *You can make the dressing a day ahead of time, and store in the fridge to let the flavors meld.*

Servings: 4

Cooking Times

Total Time: 10 minutes

Nutrition Facts (per serving)

Calories 235, 82

Total Fat 17,65g 27%

Total Carbohydrates 10,99g 4%

Fiber 1,65g 7%

Protein 9,84g 20%

Herb Baked Salmon Fillets

Ingredients

2 lbs. salmon fillets

1/2 cup chopped fresh mushrooms

1/2 cup chopped green onions

4 oz. butter

4 Tbsp. coconut oil

1/2 cup tamari soy sauce

1 tsp. minced garlic

1/4 tsp. thyme

1/2 tsp. rosemary

1/4 tsp. tarragon

1/2 tsp. ground ginger

1/2 tsp. basil

1 tsp. oregano leaves

Directions

1. Preheat oven to 350 degrees F. Line a large baking pan with foil.
2. Cut salmon filet in pieces. Put the salmon into the ziploc bag with the tamari sauce, sesame oil and spices sauce mixture. Refrigerate the salmon and marinade it for 4 hours.
3. Put the salmon in a baking pan and bake fillets for 10-15 minutes.

4. Melt the butter. Add the chopped fresh mushrooms and green onion to it, and mix. Remove the salmon from the oven, and pour the butter mixture over the salmon fillets, making sure each fillet gets covered.
5. Bake for about 10 minutes more. Serve immediately.

Servings: 6

Cooking Times

Inactive Time: 4 hours

Total Time: 35 minutes

Nutrition Facts (per serving)

Calories 449, 77

Total Fat 34,11g 52%

Total Carbohydrates 2,77g <1%

Fiber 0,72g 3%

Protein 33,19g 66%

Beef Cabbage Parsley Soup

Ingredients

1 lb. beef shank

1/2 head cabbage, chopped

6 tsp. fresh parsley (chopped)

2 zucchini, cubed

1 tomato, quartered

1 onion, chopped

4 cloves garlic, minced

1 Tbsp. salt

1/4 tsp. ground cumin

2 Tbsp. fresh lime juice

Directions

1. In a large pot over low heat combine the beef, tomato, zucchini, onion, cabbage, garlic, 5 teaspoons parsley, salt and cumin.

2. Add water to cover and stir well. Cover lid and cook for 2 hours.

3. Remove lid, stir, and simmer for another 1 hour with lid off.

4. Just before eating, squeeze in fresh lime juice to taste and sprinkle with remaining parsley.

5. Serve hot.

Servings: 8

Cooking Times

Total Time: 2 hours and 5 minutes

Nutrition Facts (per serving)

Calories 129, 83

Total Fat 2,35g

Total Carbohydrates 13,28g

Fiber 2,08g

Protein 14,11g

Boneless Lamb Stew

Ingredients

2 lbs. boneless lamb meat, cubed

1 cup red onion, chopped

2 whole celery stalks, diced

4 cloves garlic, minced

1 cup tomato juice

2 Tbsp. extra virgin coconut oil

1 cup lime juice (freshly squeezed)

1 bay leaf

1 tsp. ground cinnamon

1 tsp. ground nutmeg

Fresh parsley, chopped for topping

Sea salt and freshly ground black pepper, to taste

Directions

1. Put the lamb in a glass bowl and season with the salt, pepper, cinnamon, and nutmeg. Place in refrigerator for up to 24 hours.

2. In a large casserole, heat the coconut oil over medium heat. Add pieces of lamb and brown on all sides.

3. Once browned, add the onion, garlic and celery. Cook for about five minutes, stirring often, until vegetables start to soften.

4. Add the tomato juice, lime juice and bay leaf; stir till mixture begins to boil.

5. Reduce the heat to low and cook for about 2 hours.

6. Serve hot with fresh chopped parsley.

Servings: 6

Cooking Times

Total Time: 2 hours and 10 minutes

Nutrition Facts (per serving)

Calories 250, 3

Total Fat 11,82g 18%

Total Carbohydrates 6,86g 2%

Fiber 1,67g 7%

Protein 21,68g 43%

Butternut Squash Soup

Ingredients

3 lbs. butternut squash

4 cloves garlic, minced

1 cup yellow onion, sliced

1 cup coconut milk

2 tsp. olive oil

1 bay leaf

2 cup water

1/2 tsp. salt and pepper (per taste)

coconut oil or olive oil for greasing

Directions

1. Preheat oven to 450° F.
2. On a greased baking sheet, place the squash and onion with half oil and salt. Roast in a single layer about 25-30 minutes.
3. Transfer the vegetables to a large saucepan with olive oil and cook over HIGH heat for 3-5 minutes. Stir often.
4. Add garlic and cook for another 30 seconds. Add the water, bay leaf and coconut milk; bring to a boil.
5. Reduce heat to MEDIUM-LOW, cover and simmer for 10 minutes more.
6. At the end, remove bay leaf and transfer squash mixture to a blender. Puree until smooth. Add salt and pepper to taste.
7. Ladle to bowls and serve hot.

Servings: 10

Cooking Times

Total Time: 55 minutes

Nutrition Facts (per serving)

Calories 120, 27

Total Fat 7,12g 11%

Total Carbohydrates 12,74g 4%

Fiber 2,3g 9%

Protein 3,48g 7%

Creamy Chicken Salad

Ingredients

Salad ingredients

2 cups diced, cooked chicken

1/2 cup sliced green onion

1/4 cup parsley, chopped

1/2 cup diced celery

Dressing ingredients

4 oz. mayonnaise

2 oz. blue cream cheese, softened

1 tsp. dried tarragon

1/2 tsp. dried thyme

salt and pepper to taste

Directions

1. In a bowl, whisk cream cheese and mayonnaise until smooth.
2. Add the spices and continue to whisk.
3. Combine the salad ingredients and add dressing to taste, mixing to coat all the ingredients.
4. Serve immediately.

Servings: 4

Cooking Times

Total Time: 10 minutes

Nutrition Facts (per serving)

Calories 250, 36

Total Fat 12,23g 19%

Total Carbohydrates 9,77g 3%

Fiber 0,78g 3%

Protein 24,74g 49%

Duck Breast with Balsamic Vinegar

Ingredients

1 lb. duck breasts

4 Tbsp. duck fat (or lark)

4 green onions (chopped)

1 tsp. fresh ginger grated

1/2 Tbsp. lime juice

Marjoram to taste

2 Tbsp. coconut oil

2 Tbsp. apple cider vinegar

salt and freshly ground pepper to taste

Directions

1. In a frying pan add 1 tablespoon coconut oil and add the duck breast. Sauté it at high heat about 3-4 minutes.
2. In a deep saucepan add the duck fat, and add the duck meat. Cook for 3 hours about. Add the chopped green onions in the last 30 minutes of the cooking process.
3. Remove green onion and duck breast from the heat, and place them in a separate dish to cool down. Sprinkle the marjoram, balsamic vinegar and the lime juice. Serve hot.

Servings: 4

Nutrition Facts (per serving)

Calories 471, 59

Total Fat 46,68g 72%

Total Carbohydrates 2,76g <1%

Fiber 0,42g 2%

Protein 10,11g 20%

Hot Mexican Meatballs

Ingredients

1 lb. ground beef (92% lean)

4 oz. white onion, minced

4 oz. Monterey Jack cheese with spicy peppers

1 Tbsp. butter

3 cloves garlic

1 1 tsp. chili powder

1 1 tsp. ground cumin

1 tsp. ground coriander

1 egg

sea salt and freshly ground pepper to taste

Directions

1. Preheat oven to 350 degrees.
2. In a frying pan, sauté onions in butter until translucent. Set aside
3. Shred and mince the Monterey Jack cheese with spicy peppers. Set aside.
4. In a mixing bowl, whisk egg with ricotta cheese. Add the spices, salt, and pepper and mix.
5. Add onions and minced Monterey Jack cheese with spicy peppers. Mix well.
6. Add beef and mix until all ingredients are combined.
7. Roll the meat mix into a ball.
8. Place the meatballs on a cookie sheet, and bake about 20 minutes.
9. Serve hot.

Servings: 6

Cooking Times

Total Time: 35 minutes

Nutrition Facts (per serving)

Calories 321, 28

Total Fat 25,25g 39%

Total Carbohydrates 2,94g <1%

Fiber 0,9g 4%

Protein 19,54g 39%

Lamb Cutlets with Garlic Sauce

Ingredients

4 lbs. lamb cutlets

1 small head of garlic, cloves peeled

2 Tbsp. apple cider vinegar

1/2 cup water

1/4 cup extra virgin olive oil

pinch salt and black ground pepper to taste

Directions

1. Crush the garlic cloves thoroughly in a mortar. In a bowl, add the vinegar and water and mix it well with the crushed garlic. Set aside.
2. In a large frying pan, pour the olive oil and fry the lamb cutlets until nicely brown.
3. Add the garlic mixture and let it cook gently for about 10 minutes.
4. Shake the frying pan to spread the garlic mixture evenly over the lamb.
5. Season with salt and black pepper to taste. Serve.

Servings: 10

Cooking Times

Total Time: 40 minutes

Nutrition Facts (per serving)

Calories 416, 68

Total Fat 28,76g 44%

Total Carbohydrates 0,16g <1%

Fiber 0,01g <1%

Protein 36,68g 73%

Almond Bread

Ingredients

2 eggs

1 cup almond butter, unsalted

3/4 cup almond flour

1 Tbsp. cinnamon

1 tsp. pure vanilla extract

1/4 tsp. baking soda

2 Tbsp. liquid Stevia

1/2 tsp. sea salt

Directions

1. Preheat oven to 340F degrees.
2. In a deep bowl whisk eggs, almond butter, honey, Stevia and vanilla. Add in salt, cinnamon and baking soda. Stir until all ingredients are well combined.
3. Pour dough in a greased baking pan. Bake for 12-15 minutes.
4. Once ready, let cool on a wire rack. Slice and serve.

Servings: 8

Cooking Times

Total Time: 25 minutes

Nutrition Facts (per serving)

Calories 208, 06

Total Fat 16,7g 26%

Total Carbohydrates 7,64g 3%

Fiber 3,63g 15%

Protein 7,7g 15%

Slow Cooker Buffalo Chicken

Ingredients

3 Tbsp. butter

6 frozen chicken breasts

1 bottle of your favorite cayenne peppers sauce

1 cup of your favorite garlic sauce

Directions

1. Put the chicken in the bottom of your Slow Cooker. Pour the hot sauce over chicken and sprinkle ranch over top
2. Cover the lid and cook on LOW for 6 hours.
3. Once ready, add butter, and cook on LOW uncovered for one hour more. Serve hot.

Servings: 4

Cooking Time: 6 hours and 5 minutes

Nutrition Facts (per serving)

Calories 517, 01

Total Fat 18,41g

Total Carbohydrates 2,26g

Fiber 0,37g

Protein 80,37g

Spiced Kale "Meatballs"

Ingredients

4 Tbsp. olive oil

1 cup almond flour

1 bunch of kale leaves

1 green chili, chopped

1/4 tsp. red chili powder

1/4 tsp. turmeric powder

1 tsp. cumin seed powder

1/4 tsp. ginger, minced

black salt or salt as per taste

1 tsp. cooking soda or baking soda (optional)

water for batter

Directions

1. In a bowl, mix all the ingredients together.
2. Combine and knead the batter with your finger. The consistency should be nor too thick nor too thin. Make a kale "meatballs".
3. Heat oil in a frying pan. Place a kale "meatballs" in the hot oil one by one.
4. Fry few at a time don't cluster with too many. When they get golden color from one side, turn and cook from another side.
5. Remove the fries with slotted spoon and place over absorbent napkins.
6. Serve hot.

Servings: 8

Cooking Times

Total Time: 25 minutes

Nutrition Facts (per serving)

Calories 125, 94

Total Fat 6,24g 10%

Total Carbohydrates 13,01g 4%

Fiber 4,85g 19%

Protein 6,04g 12%

Spinach Soup with Almonds and Parmesan

Ingredients

1 lb. baby spinach leaves

1 leek

1 zucchini (medium)

1/4 cup parmesan cheese (grated)

4 Tbsp. olive oil

4 cups water

15 almond shivers

salt and black ground pepper to taste

Directions

1. Wash the leek and cut it into thick slices.

2. Heat the olive oil in a saucepan and cook the zucchini and leek for about 2-3 minutes.

3. Add the cleaned spinach leaves, water and a pinch of salt. Bring to the boil and let it simmer for 15 minutes.

4. Remove from the heat and place the vegetables in a food processor. Blend into a very smooth soup.

5. In a frying pan, toast the almonds. Pour the soup into bowls, sprinkle with some Parmesan cheese on top and toasted almonds.

6. Serve.

Servings: 6

Cooking Times

Total Time: 45 minutes

Nutrition Facts (per serving)

Calories 63, 42

Total Fat 3,04g

Total Carbohydrates 5,94g

Fiber 2,47g

Protein 4,84g

Stuffed Avocado with Tuna

Ingredients

2 ripe avocados, halved and pitted

1 can (15 oz.) solid white tuna packed in water, drained

2 Tbsp. mayonnaise

3 green onions, thinly sliced

1 Tbsp. cayenne paprika

1 red bell pepper, chopped

1 Tbsp. balsamic vinegar

1 pinch garlic salt and black pepper to taste

Directions

1. In a bowl, toss together tuna, mayonnaise, cayenne pepper, green onions, red pepper, and balsamic vinegar.
2. Season with pepper and salt, and then pack the avocado halves with the tuna mixture.
3. Ready! Serve and enjoy!

Servings: 4

Cooking Times

Total Time: 20 minutes

Nutrition Facts (per serving)

Calories 233, 3

Total Fat 17,77g 27%

Total Carbohydrates 13,87g 5%

Fiber 6,98g 28%

Protein 7,41g 15%

Light Cabbage Soup

Ingredients

2 1/2 cups chopped cabbage

4 garlic cloves, minced

1 Tbsp. tomato paste

1 onion, chopped

1/2 cup parsnip, chopped

1/2 cup cauliflower florets

1/2 cup chopped zucchini

1/2 tsp. basil

1/2 tsp. oregano

Salt and black pepper, to taste

4 cups water

olive oil for sautéing

Directions

1. In a frying pan, sauté onions, parsnip and garlic for 5 minutes.
2. Add in water, tomato paste, cabbage, cauliflower, basil, oregano and salt and pepper to taste.
3. Simmer for a about 5-10 minutes until all vegetables are tender. Add the zucchini and simmer for another 5 minutes.
4. Serve hot.

Servings: 4

Cooking Times

Total Time: 35 minutes

Nutrition Facts (per serving)

Calories 80, 31

Total Fat 3,08g 5%

Total Carbohydrates 9,69g 3%

Fiber 3,04g 12%

Protein 4,62g 9%

Oriental Shrimp Soup

Ingredients

12 oz. fresh shrimp, peeled and deveined

1 cup zucchini (medium, sliced)

1 onion, chopped

2 cloves garlic, minced

1 Tbsp. ginger, minced

1 pinch crushed red pepper

2 quarts water

1 cup celery (chopped)

2 cups cauliflower florets

2 Tbsp. soy sauce

1/4 tsp. ground black pepper

2 tsp. olive oil

Directions

1. In a large saucepan with over medium heat cook onion, garlic, ginger and crushed red pepper for 2 minutes.
2. Pour in water, cauliflower florets and celery and bring to a boil. Reduce heat, cover and simmer 5 minutes.
3. Stir in zucchini and shrimp, season with salt and pepper to taste; cover and cook 5 - 7 minutes.
4. Stir in soy sauce and pepper and serve.

Servings: 8

Cooking Times

Total Time: 25 minutes

Nutrition Facts (per serving)

Calories 107, 62

Total Fat 3,08g 5%

Total Carbohydrates 7,12g 2%

Fiber 1,6g 6%

Protein 12,08g 24%

Slow Cooker Beef with Dried Herbs

Ingredients

1 1/2 lbs. lean beef

2 celery ribs

1 cup beef broth

2 Tbsp. amaranth flour

2 Tbsp. almond butter

2 Tbsp. olive oil

1 tsp. mustard

2 Tbsp. fresh lemon juice

4 Tbsp. chopped parsley

salt, pepper, dried thyme, dried marjoram

Directions

1. In a bowl, toss the beef with the amaranth flour. Heat the butter and oil in a skillet; add the beef and cook, stirring, until browned.
2. In a slow cooker combine the browned beef with remaining ingredients, except lemon juice and parsley.
3. Cover and cook on LOW for 6 to 8 hours.
4. Once ready, stir in lemon juice and parsley and serve hot.

Servings: 6

Cooking Times

Total Time: 8 hours

Nutrition Facts (per serving)

Calories 387, 96

Total Fat 31,96g 49%

Total Carbohydrates 2,56g <1%

Fiber 0,2g <1%

Protein 20,96g 42%

Zucchini Soup with Crunchy Cured Ham

Ingredients

2 leeks (white part only)

12 ounces zucchinis

10 ounces summer squash

3 Tbsp. virgin olive oil

5 cups water

salt

2 slices cured ham

black pepper

Directions

1. Cut the leeks into thin slices and chop the zucchinis and summer squash into cubes.

2. In a large saucepan, heat the olive oil and add the leeks. Cook the leeks until they are soft, stirring gently.

3. Add in the chopped zucchinis and summer squash and cook them for about 5 minutes.

4. Add in water and bring to the boil for about 15 minutes.

5. Blend or process the soup in batches until smooth.

6. Season the soup to taste.

7. In a frying pan cook striped ham until crispy.

8. Divide the soup amongst the serving bowls and sprinkle with the crunchy ham strips and some black pepper.

9. Serve hot.

Servings: 4

Cooking Times

Total Time: 45 minutes

Nutrition Facts (per serving)

Calories 84, 19

Total Fat 1,89g 3%

Total Carbohydrates 8,75g 3%

Fiber 1,52g 6%

Protein 8,54g 17%

Salmon with a Walnut Crust

Ingredients

Walnuts (1/2 cup)

Dijon mustard (1/2 tablespoon)

Salmon filets (6 oz.)-2

Salt

Maple syrup (2 tablespoons, sugar free)

Dill (1/4 teaspoon)

Olive oil (1 tablespoon)

Directions

1. Set oven to 350 F.

2. Put mustard, syrup and walnuts into a processor and pulse until mixture is pasty.

3. Heat oil in a pot and place the skin side down in the pan and sear for 3 minutes.

4. Top it with walnut blend and place into a lined baking dish.

5. Bake for 8 minutes.

6. Serve.

Servings: 2

Nutrition Facts (per serving)

Calories 373

Net Carbs 3g

Fats 43g

Protein 20 g

Fiber 1g

Cheeseburger Casserole

Ingredients

Bacon (3 slices)

Cauliflower (1 ¼ cups)

Garlic powder (1/2 teaspoon)

Ketchup (2 tablespoons, no sugar)

Mayonnaise (2 tablespoons)

Cheddar cheese (4 oz.)

Ground beef (1 lb.)

Almond flour (1/2 cup)

Psyllium Husk Powder (1 tablespoon)

Onion powder (1/2 teaspoon)

Dijon mustard (1 tablespoon)

Eggs (3)

Salt

Black pepper

Directions

1. Set oven to 350 °F.

2. Place cauliflower into a processor and pulse until fine like rice. Add remaining dry ingredients except cheese.

3. Add beef and bacon in processor until combined and pasty.

4. Heat skillet and cook meat for 8 minutes then add to dry ingredients in bowl along with half of cheese. Stir to combine and line a baking dish with parchment paper.

5. Press mixture into dish and top with leftover cheese. Bake for 30 minutes on top rack.

6. Take from heat, cool and slice.

7. Serve.

Servings: 6

Nutrition Facts (per serving)

Calories 478

Net Carbs 3.6g

Fats 35.5g

Protein 32.2 g

Fiber 3.3g

Curried Coconut Chicken Fingers

Ingredients

Chicken thighs (24 oz., boneless with skin)

Pork rinds (1/2 cup, crushed)

Curry powder (2 teaspoons)

Garlic powder (1/4 teaspoon)

Salt

Black pepper

Egg (1)

Coconut (1/2 cup, shredded, unsweetened)

Coriander (1/2 teaspoon)

Onion powder (1/4 teaspoon)

For Dipping Sauce:

Sour cream (1/4 cup)

Mango extract (1 ½ teaspoons)

Garlic powder (1/2 teaspoon)

Cayenne powder (1/4 teaspoon)

Mayonnaise (1/4 cup)

Ketchup (2 tablespoons, sugar free)

Red pepper flakes (1 ½ teaspoons)

Ground ginger (1/2 teaspoon)

Liquid Stevia (7 drops)

Directions

1. Set oven to 400 °F.

2. Beat egg in a bowl and slice chicken into strips.

3. Combine spices, pork rind and coconut in another bowl. Coat with egg and then in dry mix.

4. Place onto a lined baking sheet and bake for 15 minutes and turn over; bake for an additional 20 minutes.

5. Combine all ingredients for dipping sauce in a bowl and serve with chicken.

Servings: 6

Nutrition Facts (per serving)

Calories 494

Net Carbs 2.1g

Fats 39.4g

Protein 29.4 g

Fiber 1.2g

Slow Cooker Lamb Curry & Spinach

Ingredients

Coconut or olive oil (1/3 cup)

3 copped yellow onions

4 cloves garlic, peeled and minced

2cm piece of ginger, peeled and grated

Ground cumin (2 teaspoons)

Cayenne pepper (1 1/2 teaspoons).

Ground turmeric (1 1/2 teaspoons).

Beef stock, high quality (2 cups)

Leg of lamb, cut into 2cm cubes (53 oz.)

Salt

Baby spinach (6 cups)

Plain full-fat yogurt (2 cups)

Directions

1. In a large frying pan over medium-high heat, warm oil. Add onions and garlic, and sauté until golden, about 5 minutes. Stir in ginger, cumin, cayenne, and turmeric and sauté until fragrant, or for about 30 seconds.

2. Pour in broth scraping up the browned bits on the bottom. When broth comes to a boil, remove pan from heat.

3. Put lamb in a slow cooker, and sprinkle with 1 tbsp. salt. Add contents of frying pan. Cover and cook on high-heat setting for 4 hours or low-heat setting for 8 hours.

4. Add baby spinach to pot and cook, stirring occasionally, until spinach is wilted, about 5 minutes. Just before serving, stir in 1 1/3 cups yogurt. Season to taste with salt.

Servings: 5

Nutrition Facts (per serving)

Calories- 304

Carbs- 5.5g

Protein- 32.85g

Fats- 16.32g

Curried Madras Lamb

Ingredients

8 Fatty lamb chops

Coconut Milk (6 tablespoons)

2 cups water

Red Curry Paste (3 tablespoons)

Thai fish sauce (2 tablespoons)

Dried onion flakes (1 tablespoon)

Dried Thai or fresh red chilies (2 tablespoons)

Xylitol (1 tablespoon)

Ground cumin (1 tablespoon)

Ground coriander (1 tablespoon)

Ground cloves (1/8 teaspoon)

Ground nutmeg (1/8 teaspoon)

Ground ginger (1 tablespoon)

To Serve:

Coconut milk powder (2 tablespoons)

Red curry paste (1 tablespoons)

Xylitol (2 tablespoons)

1/4 cup cashews, roughly chopped

1/4 cup fresh cilantro, chopped

Directions

1. Place the raw lamb chops in a large slow cooker.

2. Add the 6 tbsp. coconut milk, water, 3 tbsp. red curry paste, fish sauce, onion flakes, chilies, 1 tbsp. Xylitol, cumin, coriander, cloves, nutmeg, and ginger. Cover and cook on high for about 5 hours (or low for 8).

3. Just before serving, scoop out the meat to another dish. Then whisk into the sauce the 2 tbsp. coconut milk powder, 1 tbsp. curry paste, 2 tbsp. sweetener, and 1/4 tsp. xanthan gum (if using).

4. Break the meat into pieces and stir into the sauce, along with the chopped cashews. Garnish with chopped coriander before serving

Servings: 5

Nutrition Facts (per serving)

Calories- 190

Carbs- 4g

Protein- 18g

Fats- 11g

Seafood Stew

Ingredients

Olive oil (1 tablespoon)

2 onions, diced

4 stalks celery, chopped

4 garlic cloves, minced

Dried oregano (1 teaspoon)

Ground black pepper (1/2 teaspoon)

Tomato paste (1 tablespoon)

Flour (1 tablespoon)

3 cups chicken stock

1 can tomato, onion and chili mix

1 -2 cup tomato cocktail juice

4 chicken breasts cut into bite size pieces

2 packets mixed frozen seafood, you can add extra

mussels in at the end

2 peppers (red and green)

1 jalapeno pepper, chopped

1/4cup parsley, chopped

Chili powder (1 teaspoon)

1 pinch cayenne pepper

Butter (1 tablespoon)

Directions

1. In a large pan heat the olive oil and fry onions and celery

2. Add garlic, oregano, peppercorns.

3. Stir in tomato paste and almond flour and cook another minute.

4. Add chicken stock, tomatoes and tomato juice and bring to a boil. Continue to cook for about 3-5 more minutes. Remove from heat and transfer mixture to slow cooker.

5. Add chicken and stir to combine. Cover and cook on high for 3 hours or low for 6 hours.

6. Stir in mixed bags of frozen and parsley. Cover and cook on high for 30 minutes

Servings: 5

Nutrition Facts (per serving)

Calories- 177

Carbs- 15g

Protein- 21g

Fats- 4g

Slow Cooker Thai Fish Curry

Ingredients

Coconut oil (1 tablespoon)

Green Thai curry paste (1/2 tablespoons)

8-10 spring onions

2 garlic cloves, crushed

1 Thai red chili, deseeded if you like, and thinly sliced

Turmeric (1 teaspoon)

Chicken stock (160ml)

1½ cups coconut milk

2.5cm piece of fresh ginger, peeled and sliced

Xylitol (2 teaspoons)

Juice of 1 lime, plus extra to taste

Fish sauce (1 teaspoon)

700g boneless, skinless white fish, such as cod, hake or halibut cut into large chunks

freshly ground black pepper

chopped coriander leaves, to serve

Directions

1. Fry Spring onions, garlic and chilies then stir in green Thai Curry Paste and then sprinkle over the turmeric.

2. Add the stock, coconut milk, ginger, Xylitol and juice from a fresh lime and season with pepper. Bring to the boil, stirring to dissolve the paste and xylitol, and then pour the mixture into the slow cooker.

3. Cover the cooker with the lid and cook on HIGH for 1 hour until the flavors are well blended. Add the fish sauce, if using, and add a little more xylitol and fresh lime juice, if you like.

4. Switch the cooker to LOW. Add the fish, re-cover and cook until the fish is cooked through and flakes easily.

5. Sprinkle with coriander and lime zest and sliced red chilies.

Servings: 5

Nutrition Facts (per serving)

Calories- 312

Carbs- 20g

Protein- 24g

Fats- 15g

Smoky Pork Cassoulet

Ingredients

1 pack bacon, fried and then crumbled

Chopped onion (2 cups)

Dried thyme (1 teaspoon)

Dried rosemary (1/2 teaspoon)

3 garlic cloves, crushed

Salt (1/2 teaspoon)

Freshly ground black pepper (1/2 teaspoon)

2 cans diced tomatoes, drained

500g boneless pork loin roast, trimmed and cut into 2cm cubes

250g smoked sausage, cut into 1cm cubes

Finely shredded fresh Parmesan cheese (8 teaspoons)

Chopped fresh flat-leaf parsley (8 teaspoons)

Directions

1. Fry bacon onion, thyme, rosemary, and garlic, then add salt, pepper, and tomatoes; bring to a boil.

2. Remove from heat.

3. Place all ingredients in the slow cooker, alternating the meat with the tomato sauce until finished. Cover and cook on low for 5 hours. Sprinkle with Parmesan cheese and parsley when cooked

Servings: 4

Nutrition Facts (per serving)

Calories- 258

Carbs- 10.8g

Protein- 27g

Fats- 12.6g

Sage and Orange Glazed Duck

Ingredients

Butter (2 tablespoons)

Swerve (1 tablespoon)

Sage (1/4 teaspoon)

Duck breast (6 oz.)

Heavy cream (1 tablespoon)

Orange extract (1/2 teaspoon)

Spinach (1 cup)

Directions

1. Use knife to score the skin of the duck and season with black pepper and salt.

2. Add Swerve and butter to a pot and cook until slightly golden then add extract and sage. Cook until butter has darkened.

3. In another pot, place chicken breast with skin side down and place over a medium flame and cook until skin is crisp.

4. Flip over and add cream to sage mixture and pour over duck. Cook until duck is done.

5. Add spinach to pot and cook until wilted.

6. Serve.

Servings: 1

Nutrition Facts (per serving)

Calories 798

Net Carbs 0g

Fats 71g

Protein 36 g

Fiber 1g

Chicken Pot Pie

Ingredients

For filling:

Bacon (5 slices)

Garlic powder (1 teaspoon)

Cream cheese (8 oz.)

Spinach (6 cups)

Salt

Chicken thighs (6, boneless and skinless)

Onion powder (1 teaspoon)

Celery seed (3/4 teaspoon)

Cheddar cheese (4 oz.)

Chicken broth (1/4 cup)

For crust:

Psyllium Husk Powder (3 tablespoons)

Eggs (1)

Cheddar cheese (1/4 cup)

Garlic powder (1/4 teaspoon)

Salt

Almond flour (1/3 cup)

Butter (3 tablespoons)

Cream cheese (1/4 cup)

Paprika (1/2 teaspoon)

Onion powder (1/4 teaspoon)

Black pepper

Directions

1. Cube chicken and season with black pepper and salt.

2. Set oven to 375 F.

3. Use spices to season chicken and place into an oven proof skillet and place onto fire and cook until golden on the outside. Add bacon to pan and cook until golden.

4. Add broth to pan along with cheeses and stir to combine. Put in spinach in pan and cook until wilted.

5. Combine dry ingredients for crust in a bowl and add cheddar and cream cheese to a microwave safe dish and then add cheese and combine. Add mixture to dry ingredients and mix together.

6. Form crust, stir ingredients in pot and top with crust and use fork to pierce crust all over.

7. Bake for 15 minutes, take from oven and cool.

8. Serve.

Servings: 8

Nutrition Facts (per serving)

Calories 434

Net Carbs 3.4g

Fats 35.6g

Protein 20.4 g

Fiber 3.6g

Chicken Parmesan

Ingredients

For Chicken:

Chicken breasts (3)

Mozzarella cheese (1 cup)

Salt

Black pepper

For coating:

Flaxseed meal (1/4 cup)

Oregano (1 teaspoon)

Black pepper (1/2 teaspoon)

Garlic powder (1/2 teaspoon)

Egg (1)

Pork rinds (2.5 oz.)

Parmesan cheese (1/2 cup)

Salt (1/2 teaspoon)

Red pepper flakes (1/4 teaspoon)

Paprika (2 teaspoons)

Chicken broth (1 ½ teaspoons)

For Sauce:

Tomato sauce (1 cup, low carb)

Garlic (2 cloves)

Salt

Olive oil (1/2 cup)

Oregano (1/2 teaspoon)

Black pepper

Directions

1. Add flax meal, spices, pork rinds and parmesan cheese in a processor and grind until combined.
2. Pound chicken breast and whisk egg with broth in a container. Add all ingredients for sauce to a pan stir and put over a low flame to cook.
3. Dip chicken in egg and then coat with dry mixture.
4. Heat oil in a pan and fry chicken then transfer to a casserole dish. Top with sauce and mozzarella and bake for 10 minutes.
5. Serve.

Servings: 4

Nutrition Facts (per serving)

Calories 646

Net Carbs 4g

Fats 46.8g

Protein 49.3g

Fiber 2.8g

Bell Peppers Stuffed Korean Beef

Ingredients

Ground beef (1 lb.)

Spring onions (2, sliced)

Ginger (2 teaspoons, diced)

Eggs (8)

Bell peppers (2, cut in half)

Garlic (2 teaspoons, diced)

Salt

Black pepper

For Sauce:

Rice wine vinegar (1 ½ tablespoons)

Chili paste (1 tablespoon)

Apricot preserves (1/3 cup, sugar free)

Ketchup (1 tablespoon, low sugar)

Soy sauce (1 tablespoon)

Directions

1. Season beef with pepper and salt and start cooking over a medium flame until browned. Add ginger and garlic and stir together.

2. Push beef to one side and put in spring onions, cook for 2 minutes then stir together with beef. Take from flame and put aside.

3. Add all sauce ingredients to a pan and cook for 3 minutes then add half to beef.

4. Stir sauce and beef together and use to stuff peppers.

5. Set oven to 350 F and bake for 15 minutes.

6. Top with reserved sauce and serve.

Servings: 4

Nutrition Facts (per serving)

Calories 470

Net Carbs 6.3g

Fats 35g

Protein 32.3g

Fiber 5.3g

Creamy Tarragon Chicken

Ingredients

Chicken breast (5 oz.)

Onion (1/4, sliced)

Chicken broth (1/2 cup)

Grain mustard (1 teaspoon)

Salt

Olive oil (1 tablespoon)

Mushrooms (3 oz.)

Heavy cream (1/4 cup)

Tarragon (1/2 teaspoon, dried)

Black pepper

Directions

1. Cube chicken and season with pepper and salt.

2. Heat oil in a pan and sauté chicken for 6 minutes until golden all over. Take from pan and put aside.

3. Add mushrooms and cook for 3 minutes until golden then add onion and cook for 3 minutes until soft and translucent.

4. Add broth and bring to a boil for 4 minutes then add remaining ingredients and adjust black pepper and salt to taste.

5. Return chicken to sauce in pan and cook for 5 minutes.

6. Serve.

Servings: 1

Nutrition Facts (per serving)

Calories 490

Net Carbs 5g

Fats 40g

Protein 32 g

Fiber 1g

Beanless Chili con Carne

Ingredients

Ground beef (1 lb.)

Green pepper (1, chopped)

Onion (1, chopped)

Curry powder (2 tablespoons)

Cumin (2 tablespoons)

Coconut oil (1 tablespoon)

Onion powder (1 teaspoon)

Black pepper (1 teaspoon)

Italian sausage (1 lb., spicy)

Yellow pepper (1, chopped)

Tomato sauce (16 oz.)

Chili powder (2 tablespoons)

Garlic (1 tablespoon, diced)

Butter (1 tablespoon)

Salt (1 teaspoon)

Directions

1. Heat oil and butter in a pan, heat thoroughly and add garlic, onions and bell peppers. Cook for 3 minutes then add beef and sausage.

2. Cook for 5 minutes until browned then add onion and chili powder. Stir to combine and add tomato sauce. Lower flame and cook for 20 minutes.

3. Add cumin and curry, stir and cook for 45 minutes or until chili thickens to your liking.

4. Serve.

Servings: 5

Nutrition Facts (per serving)

Calories 415

Net Carbs 6g

Fats 25g

Protein 146 g

Fiber 51g

Seared Ribeye Steak

Ingredients

Ribeye steaks (2 medium)

Salt

Black pepper

Bacon fat (3 tablespoons)

Directions

1. Set oven to 250 °F.
2. Place a wire rack over a baking sheet and place steaks on rack.
3. Use pepper and salt to season steaks and bake until steak's internal temperature is 123 °F.
4. Melt fat in a cast iron pan until it is extremely hot then transfer steaks to pot and sear on both sides.
5. Let steaks sit for a few minutes before slicing.
6. Serve.

Servings: 5

Nutrition Facts (per serving)

Calories 430

Net Carbs 0g

Fats 31.7g

Protein 30.3 g

Fiber 0g

Italian Fish Stew

Ingredients

4 200g Kingklip fish fillets

2 onions, finely chopped

4 garlic cloves, minced

2 tins peeled, chopped tomato

4 tbsp. tomato paste

250ml white wine

½ tsp. parsley, chopped

¼ tsp. dried oregano

salt and pepper to taste

½ cup olive oil

1 cup water

Directions

1. Preheat oven to 360C
2. Sauté onion and garlic on a pot then add tinned tomatoes and tomato paste and stir.
3. Pour the wine, parsley, oregano, salt, pepper, and water. Stir well and bring to a simmer.
4. Let it simmer for 10-15 minutes to reduce and thicken.
5. Meanwhile, place your fish in baking dish.
6. When sauce is nice and thick, pour it over fish and sprinkle with a little extra oregano.
7. Cover the dish with foil and place in the oven to cook for 20 minutes.
8. Take foil off and return to oven uncovered and cook for another 10 minutes.

Tip: If the sauce is a little runny when fish comes out, place sauce in another pot and put on heat to reduce a little more. Then pour back over fish.

Nutritional Info (per serving)

Calories: 315

Net Carbs: 12

Fat: 8g

Protein: 37g

Chicken Stir-Fry

Ingredients

4 chicken breasts (butterfly), marinate in egg white overnight

 2 cups red pepper

2 cups mange tout

2 cups grated carrot

2 cups broccoli

2 cups almonds

2 cloves of garlic

½ tsp. ginger

2 tbsp. soya sauce

125ml chicken stock.

2 tbsp. coconut oil

Directions

1. Heat coconut oil in a pan over medium fire. Sauté the garlic and ginger until fragrant.
2. Cook the chicken breast in the oil and then add the vegetables. Toss and cook until almost done.
3. Add 2 tbsp. soya sauce and 125ml chicken stock. Allow to simmer uncovered until the broth evaporates.

Nutritional Info
Calories: 186

Net Carbs: 4g

Fat: 11g

Protein: 17g

Pan Fried Hake

Ingredients

1 tbsp. olive oil

Salt and pepper to taste

1 250g Hake fillet

fresh lemon wedges

Directions

1. Heat the olive oil in a large frying pan over medium-high heat.
2. Pat the fish dry with kitchen paper towel and then season with salt and pepper on both sides.
3. Fry the fish for about 4-5 minutes on each side, depending on their thickness, or until they have a golden crust and the flesh flakes away easily with a fork.

Nutritional Info (per serving)

Calories: 170

Net Carbs: 7g

Fat: 8g

Protein: 18g

Creamed Spinach

Ingredients

2 cups spinach

½ small onion, chopped

¼ cup water

½ stock cube

1 clove of garlic, chopped

½ cup heavy cream

2 tbsp. butter

salt and pepper to taste

Directions

1. Place spinach and onion to a pan with water and heat over medium-high fire.
2. Add stock cube and garlic and allow to steam for 8-10 minutes or until all the water has evaporated and the spinach is very soft.
3. Pour in the heavy cream and butter and then season with salt and pepper. Cooking until it thickens.
4. Using a hand-held blender blitz the spinach until fairly smooth.
5. Serve while hot

Nutritional Info (1/2 cup)

Calories: 200

Net Carbs: 3g

Fat: 23g

Protein: 7g

Chicken and Mushroom Stew

Ingredients

8 pcs. chicken thighs

4 tbsp. butter

3 cloves garlic, minced

6 cups mushrooms

1 cup chicken stock

½ tsp. dried thyme

½ tsp. dried oregano

½ tsp. dried basil

¼ cup heavy cream

½ cup parmesan cheese, grated

1 tbsp. whole-grain mustard

Directions

1. Preheat oven to 400F
2. Season chicken thighs with salt and pepper
3. Heat an oven-proof pan over medium fire and melt 2 tbsp. of butter.
4. Add the chicken, skin-side down, and fry both sides until golden brown, or about 2-3 minutes per side. Set aside.
5. Melt remaining 2 tbsp. butter. Add garlic, thyme, oregano and basil and mushrooms, and cook, stirring occasionally. Cook until browned, about 5-6 minutes, season with salt and pepper, to taste.
6. Stir in chicken stock, then chicken back to the pan.
7. Pour everything into a baking dish with the chicken.
8. Place into oven and roast until completely cooked through for about 25-30 minutes. Set aside chicken.
9. Transfer sauces back into the original pan.

10. Stir in heavy cream, parmesan cheese and mustard. Bring to a boil; reduce heat and simmer until slightly reduced, about 5 minutes.
11. Serve chicken immediately, topped with mushroom mixture.

Nutritional Info (1 serving)

Calories: 203

Net Carbs: 9g

Fat: 3g

Protein: 28g

Beef Shin Stew

Ingredients

2 lb. quality shin of beef

4 tbsp. olive oil

2 red onions, peeled and roughly chopped

3 pcs. carrots, peeled and roughly chopped

3 sticks celery, trimmed and roughly chopped

4 cloves garlic, unpeeled

a few sprigs of fresh rosemary

2 bay leaves

2 cups mushrooms

2 cups baby marrows

salt and pepper to taste

1 tbsp. psyllium husk

2 cans 400 g tomatoes

⅔ bottle red wine

Directions

1. Preheat your oven to 360F
2. In a heavy-bottomed oven-proof saucepan, heat olive oil and sauté the onions, carrots, celery, garlic, herbs, and mushrooms for 5 minutes until softened slightly.
3. Meanwhile, toss the pieces of beef in the psyllium husk, shaking off any excess.
4. Add the meat to the pan and stir everything together.
5. Add the tomatoes, wine and a pinch of salt and pepper and gently bring to the boil.

6. Turn off heat then cover the sauce pan with a double-thickness piece of tinfoil and a lid and place in oven to cook for 3 hours or until the beef is meltingly tender and can be broken up with a spoon.
7. Taste and check the seasoning remove the rosemary sprigs and serve hot.

Nutritional Info (1 serving)

Calories: 315

Net Carbs: 7g

Fat: 7g

Protein: 20g

Bacon, Beef Sausage and Broccoli Casserole

Ingredients

500 g beef sausage

1/2 head of broccoli

8 slices of bacon

1/2 cup of cream

1 tbsp. Dijon mustard

100 g grated cheddar cheese

Directions

1. Preheat oven to 350F
2. Slice the sausage and place in a small baking dish.
3. Slice the bacon and add to the sausage.
4. Break the broccoli into florets and arrange between the meat.
5. Mix the cream and mustard in a bowl and pour it all over the casserole, then top with the cheese.
6. Bake in the oven for 35 minutes.

Nutritional Info (1 serving)

Calories: 300

Net Carbs: 3g

Fat: 25g

Protein: 20g

Creamy Haddock

Ingredients

150g smoked haddock

100ml boiling water

1 tbsp. butter

50ml cream

2 cups spinach

Directions

1. Heat a saucepan over medium fire.
2. Mix the boiling water with cream and butter in a bowl.
3. Place haddock and sauce in the pan and leave to boil until the water evaporates, leaving a creamy, butter sauce behind.
4. Serve haddock, covered with the sauce on fresh or wilted spinach.

Nutritional Info (1 serving)

Calories: 281

Net Carbs: 15g

Fat: 10g

Protein: 18g

Cauliflower Bake

Ingredients

4 slices of bacon

2 cups broccoli

2 cups cauliflower

2 cups mushrooms

1 green pepper

1 onion

200ml cream

120g cheese, grated

2 tbsp. olive oil

Directions

1. Preheat oven at 360F.
2. Steam or cook the cauliflower and broccoli until tender then transfer in an oven-proof dish.
3. Fry the bacon slices, with the mushrooms, green pepper and onion in 2 tbsp. olive oil.
4. Pour the fried bacon and mushrooms on top of cauliflower.
5. In a bowl, whisk 4 eggs with the cream and season to taste and pour over cauliflower or broccoli.
6. Place in the oven to cook for 25 minutes. Take out of the oven and sprinkle with grated cheese.
7. Place back in the oven and cook for another 5 minutes.

Nutritional Info (1 serving)

Calories: 100

Net Carbs: 7g

Fat: 6g

Protein: 4g

Caulicake

Ingredients

600 g cauliflower florets

1 onion, chopped

3 cloves of garlic, finely chopped

1 tsp. turmeric

100g parmesan cheese, finely grated

100g mature white cheddar cheese, coarsely grated

8 eggs

1-2 tsp. salt

2 tbsp. psyllium husk

1 cup of cream

1 tbsp. coconut oil

sesame seeds

olive oil

Directions

1. Preheat oven at 360F
2. Steam the cauliflower. Keep half of it whole and mash the rest.
3. Sauté the onion, garlic, turmeric in the coconut oil until soft. Set aside.
4. In a separate bowl, whisk the eggs. Add the cream, cheese, salt, and psyllium husk.
5. Combine the cauliflower, whole and mashed with the sautéed onions and egg mixture in a bowl.
6. Line a spring-form baking tin with greased baking paper and sprinkle with sesame seeds. Place the pan onto a baking tray.

7. Pour in the cauliflower mix and bake in the oven for 40 minutes.
8. As soon as it comes out of the oven, lightly prick the surface all over with a fork and drizzle with olive oil.

Nutritional Info (1 serving)

Calories: 160

Net Carbs: 5g

Fat: 11g

Protein: 8g

Burger Patties

Ingredients

500g ground beef

1 small onion, finely chopped

1 red pepper, chopped

¼ cup cheese, grated

1 carrot, grated

1 baby marrow, grated

1 tsp. ginger, grated

1 tsp. crushed garlic

2 eggs

2 tbsp. almond flour

1 tsp. parsley, minced

1 tsp. coriander

Salt and pepper to take

Directions

1. Mix all ingredients together in a bowl.
2. Form the mixture into balls and flatten into patties.
3. Roll the patties in almond flour and leave to firm in the fridge for around 30 minutes. This will help to keep the patties from falling apart while cooking.
4. When firm, pan fry the patties in coconut oil. Make sure your oil is hot before adding patties to the pan, you need to hear that oil sizzle. If the oil is not hot, the patty will stick to the pan and fall apart while cooking.
5. Take 1 large brown mushroom, rub with olive oil and some crushed garlic, do not salt. And bake in the oven at 360F for 15-

20mins. Place the cooked burger on top of the mushroom, add grated cheese and melt in the oven for a couple of minutes.

6. Add 1 tbsp. mayo to finely diced red onion, lettuce and tomato and place on top of burger.

Nutritional Info (1 serving)

Calories: 340

Net Carbs: 3g

Fat: 28g

Protein: 17g

Slow Cooker Oxtail Stew

Serves 10

Ingredients

1.5kg of oxtail

1 Large pack grated cabbage

1 Large pack grated carrots

2 Large onions

1 Large Bunch of celery

1 Tin of tomatoes

2 Jelly Stock Cubes

2.5 litres of water

1Tblsp Crushed garlic

1 branch Rosemary

2 Bay Leaves

Directions

1. Place all ingredients into a slow cooker and cook on medium for 9 hours.
Season with salt and pepper
2. Grate 60g cheddar cheese to finish (optional).

Chicken Hash

Ingredients

1 Tbsp. olive oil

1/4 onion finely diced

1 cups broccoli

1 cup chicken stock

50g chicken breast cooked and finely diced

½ tsp. salt

¼ tsp. black pepper

¼ cup pumpkin

Directions

1. Add all ingredients to chicken stock, cover and cook approximately 20 minutes

Tuna Fish Stew

Ingredients

1 tin tuna in water, drained

1 Tbsp. butter

¼ small onion, chopped finely

1 clove garlic, minced

1teaspoon fresh ginger, grated

½ tin tomatoes, chopped finely

1 cup spinach, chopped finely

1 small carrot, grated

1 teaspoon curry powder 1 teaspoon turmeric

½ teaspoon cayenne pepper (optional)

Salt & pepper to taste

Directions

1. Fry onion, garlic and ginger in butter.
2. Add tomatoes once onions are soft.
3. Add spices and enough water to make a stew for the spinach, carrot and tuna fish. Cook at low heat for about 15 minutes.
4. Do not overcook spinach.
5. Steam 2 cups of cauliflower, mash and add 1Tblsp of butter. Serve stew on top of the caulimash.

Ratatouille

Serves 4

Ingredients

2 large brinjals

1 large onion

2 peppers (can be green, red, yellow)

2 tins of chopped tomatoes

1 packet baby marrows

1 punnet mushrooms

1 packet spinach

500ml chicken stock

Salt & pepper

2 cloves garlic (finely chopped or pressed)

Directions

1. Finely chop all the ingredients.
2. Add all the finely chopped veggies, garlic and onion to the stock and boil on medium until the water has reduced, and the veggies have formed a thick delicious stew.
3. Serve with 150g chunky cottage cheese, 30g cheddar or 6Tblsp Parmesan Cheese

Easy Roast Tomato Sauce

Serves 10

Ingredients

10 tomatoes

Bunch of fresh basil

Garlic, bulb

Olive oil

Salt and pepper

Directions

1. Preheat oven to 190C,
2. Slice 10 tomatoes in half lengthways
3. Add a bunch of fresh basil.
4. Cut an entire bulb of garlic through the middle and place each half face up in the baking tray/dish
5. Immerse the tomatoes in olive oil and grind salt and pepper (Himalayan).
6. Roast in oven for about 1 hour and then turn the oven off for another 30 mins and leave to sit in the warm oven.
7. Remove the tomatoes and allow to cool,
8. do not mix, as you want to squeeze the flesh and pips out of the skin and discard the skin, squeeze the garlic from the cloves and throw away the casings.
9. Mash with a fork

Note: This makes THE best roast tomato sauce for pizza's meatballs or any other protein. Freeze in small Ziploc bags or plastic containers.

You can add onion, red and yellow peppers and fresh chill for more robust flavour. Use a hand blender to blitz if you want a smoother sauce.

Tender Pork & Bacon Cassoulet

Ingredients

1 pack bacon, fried and then crumbled

Chopped onion (2 cups)

Dried thyme (1 teaspoon)

Dried rosemary (1/2 teaspoon)

3 garlic cloves, crushed

Salt (1/2 teaspoon)

Freshly ground black pepper (1/2 teaspoon)

2 cans diced tomatoes, drained

500g boneless pork loin roast, trimmed and cut into 2cm cubes

250g smoked sausage, cut into 1cm cubes

Finely shredded fresh Parmesan cheese (8 teaspoons)

Chopped fresh flat-leaf parsley (8 teaspoons)

Directions

1. Fry bacon onion, thyme, rosemary, and garlic, then add salt, pepper, and tomatoes; bring to a boil.
2. Remove from heat.
3. Place all ingredients in the slow cooker, alternating the meat with the tomato sauce until finished. Cover and cook on low for 5 hours. Sprinkle with Parmesan cheese and parsley when cooked

Servings: 4

Nutrition Facts (per serving)

Calories- 258

Carbs- 10.8g

Protein- 27g

Fats- 12.6g

Lamb Cutlets with Garlic Sauce

Serves 6

Ingredients

4 lbs. lamb cutlets

1 small head of garlic, cloves peeled

2 Tbsp. apple cider vinegar

1/2 cup water

1/4 cup extra virgin olive oil

pinch salt and black ground pepper to taste

Directions

1. Crush the garlic cloves thoroughly in a mortar. In a bowl, add the vinegar and water and mix it well with the crushed garlic. Set aside.
2. In a large frying pan, pour the olive oil and fry the lamb cutlets until nicely brown.
3. Add the garlic mixture and let it cook gently for about 10 minutes.
4. Shake the frying pan to spread the garlic mixture evenly over the lamb.
5. Season with salt and black pepper to taste. Serve.

Cooking Times: 40 minutes

Amount Per Serving

Total Carbs 0,16g

Calories 416, 68

Total Fat 28,76g

Fiber 0,01g

Sugar 0,05g

Protein 36,68g

Tangy Shrimp Soup

Serves 8

Ingredients

12 oz. fresh shrimp, peeled and deveined

1 cup zucchini (medium, sliced)

1 onion, chopped

2 cloves garlic, minced

1 Tbsp. ginger, minced

1 pinch crushed red pepper

2 quarts water

1 cup celery (chopped)

2 cups cauliflower florets

2 Tbsp. soy sauce

1/4 tsp. ground black pepper

2 tsp. olive oil

Directions

1. In a large saucepan with over medium heat cook onion, garlic, ginger and crushed red pepper for 2 minutes.

2. Pour in water, cauliflower florets and celery and bring to a boil. Reduce heat, cover and simmer 5 minutes.

3. Stir in zucchini and shrimp, season with salt and pepper to taste; cover and cook 5 - 7 minutes.

4. Stir in soy sauce and pepper and serve.

Cooking Times

Total Time: 25 minutes

Amount Per Serving

Total Carbs 7,12g 2%

Calories 107, 62

Total Fat 3,08g 5%

Fiber 1,6g 6%

Sugar 3,35g

Protein 12,08g 24%

Baked Herb Salmon Fillets

Serves 6

Ingredients

2 lbs. salmon fillets

1/2 cup chopped fresh mushrooms

1/2 cup chopped green onions

4 oz. butter

4 Tbsp. coconut oil

1/2 cup tamari soy sauce

1 tsp. minced garlic

1/4 tsp. thyme

1/2 tsp. rosemary

1/4 tsp. tarragon

1/2 tsp. ground ginger

1/2 tsp. basil

1 tsp. oregano leaves

Directions

1. Preheat oven to 350 degrees F. Line a large baking pan with foil.
2. Cut salmon filet in pieces. Put the salmon into the ziploc bag with the tamari sauce, sesame oil and spices sauce mixture. Refrigerate the salmon and marinade it for 4 hours.
3. Put the salmon in a baking pan and bake fillets for 10-15 minutes.

4. Melt the butter. Add the chopped fresh mushrooms and green onion to it, and mix. Remove the salmon from the oven, and pour the butter mixture over the salmon fillets, making sure each fillet gets covered.
5. Bake for about 10 minutes more. Serve immediately.

Cooking Times

Inactive Time: 4 hours

Total Time: 35 minutes

Amount Per Serving

Total Carbs 2,77g

Calories 449, 77

Total Fat 34,11g

Fiber 0,72g

Sugar 0,79g

Protein 33,19g

Snack Recipes

Bacon & Onion Bites

Serves 12

Serving Size: 1 cookie

Ingredients

Almond flour (1 ½ cups)

Flax meal (1/3 cup)

Psyllium husk powder (1 tablespoon)

Onion powder (1 tablespoon)

1 large egg

4 slices bacon, cooked until crispy and crumbled

Sea salt (1/2 teaspoon)

Freshly ground pepper

Directions

1. Place all of the dry ingredients into a bowl (almond flour, flax meal, psyllium husk powder, onion powder, salt and pepper) and mix until well combined.
2. If you don't have onion powder, you can use dried onion flakes and blend them until powdered. Also, make sure you don't use whole psyllium husks - blend the psyllium husks until powdered if needed.
3. Add the egg and mix well using your hands.
4. Add the crumbled bacon to the dough. Process well using your hands. (Be sure to save the bacon fat from the cooking process for other uses - like some of the other fat bomb recipes in this book.)
5. Using your hand, create 12 equal balls and place them on a baking sheet lined with parchment paper.
6. Use a fork to press and flatten the dough.

Amount Per Serving

Calories: 109

Fat: 9

Parmesan Crisps

Serves 4

Serving Size: 5 crisps

Ingredients

Parmesan cheese (1 cup)

Coconut flour (4 tablespoons)

Rosemary, oregano or any herbs of choice, dried or fresh (1-2 teaspoons)

Directions

1. Preheat the oven to 350 Fahrenheit. In a small bowl, mix the coconut flour and grated parmesan cheese. Don't use finely grated or powdery parmesan cheese like you find in a canister at the supermarket, as it won't work well in this recipe. Try to find finely grated parmesan in the deli section of your supermarket, or even better, grate your own!
2. You can add any herbs you like. Oregano and rosemary work wonderfully.
3. Scoop a teaspoon of the cheese mixture onto a baking tray lined with parchment paper leaving a small gap between each. Place in the oven and cook for 10-15 minutes or until golden brown, but be careful not to burn.
4. Remove from the oven and let the crisps cool down before you remove them from the baking tray.
5. Enjoy!

Amount Per Serving

Calories: 233

Fat: 14.5

Mini Pizza Queens

Serves 6

Ingredients

14 slices Italian sausages

8 pitted black olives

3/4 cup Cream cheese

2 Tbs fresh basil, chopped

2 Tbs pesto

salt and pepper to taste

Directions

1. Dice pitted Kalamata olives and pepperoni into small pieces.
2. Mix together cream cheese, basil and pesto.
3. Add the olives and sausage slices into the cream cheese and mix again.
4. Form into balls and garnish with pepperoni, basil, and olive. Ready!!

Cooking Time: 10 minutes

Nutrition Facts (per serving)

Total Carbohydrates: 3,5g

Net Carbs: 1g

Protein: 10,4g

Total Fat: 23,43g

Calories: 261

Cheesy Bacon Balls

Serves 24

Ingredients

8 strips cooked crispy bacon, crumbled

1 cup cream cheese, softened

1/2 cup butter

4 tsp bacon fat

4 Tbsp coconut oil

1/4 cup Splenda to taste

Directions

1. In a microwave dish, combine all ingredients and melt slowly in the microwave until smooth. Set aside some crumbled bacon,
2. Pour into a dish or pan and place in the freezer until firm, about 30 minutes.
3. Before serving, remove from freezer, sprinkle with more crumbled bacon, slice and serve.

Nutrition Facts (per serving)

Total Carbohydrates: 0,5g

Dietary Fiber: 0g

Net Carbs: 0,3g

Protein: 0g

Total Fat: 15,9g

Calories: 151

Creamy Greek Balls

Serves 5

Ingredients

1 cup cream cheese, softened

1 cup butter, softened

2-3 Tbsp freshly chopped herbs (any combination of basil, thyme, oregano and/or parsley works great) or 2 teaspoons of dried herbs

4 pieces sun-dried tomatoes, drained

4 Kalamata olives, pitted and chopped

2 cloves garlic, crushed

freshly ground black pepper

1 tsp sea salt

5 Tbs parmesan cheese, finely grated

Directions

1. Mash the butter and cream cheese together with a fork and mix until well combined. Mix in the chopped sun-dried tomatoes and chopped Kalamata olives.
2. Add the freshly chopped herbs (or dried), crushed garlic and season with salt and pepper. Mix well and place in the fridge for 20-30 minutes to firm up.
3. Remove the cheese mixture from the fridge and start creating 5 balls. A spoon or an ice-cream scooper works well.
4. Place the grated parmesan cheese in a shallow dish. Roll each ball in the grated parmesan cheese and place on a plate. Eat immediately or store in the fridge in an airtight container for up to a week.
5. Enjoy!

Nutrition Facts (per serving)

Total Carbohydrates: 2,8g

Dietary Fiber: 0,24g

Net Carbs: 0,8g

Protein: 3,67g

Total Fat: 19,8g

Calories: 200

Smoked Turkey, Blue Cheese Eggs

Serves 6

Ingredients

6 eggs

2 green onions

6 oz. smoked turkey breast, chopped

1/2 cup blue cheese, crumbled

2 Tbsp. Blue cheese dressing

1/4 cup mayonnaise

2 Tbsp. hot mustard

1/2 rib celery

Directions

1. Hard boil the eggs, covered for 12 minutes.
2. In a meanwhile, chop up the smoked turkey breast and the celery.
3. Slice eggs in half lengthwise, scrape the yolks out into a bowl. Add the rest of the ingredients (except the green onions).
4. Grate the green onions over the mixture. Mix all ingredients together.
5. With the teaspoon fill every egg with the mixture.
6. Place on a serving plate and refrigerate for one hour. Ready! Serve and enjoy!

Cooking Times

Total Time: 20 minutes

Nutrition Facts (per serving)

Total Carbohydrates: 3,9g

Dietary Fiber: 0,3g

Net Carbs: 0,6g

Protein: 14g

Total Fat: 11,5g

Calories: 167

Pancetta & Eggs

Serves 4

Ingredients

4 large slices Pancetta

2 eggs, free-range

1 cup ghee, softened

2 Tbsp. mayonnaise

salt and freshly ground black pepper to taste

coconut oil for frying

Directions

1. In a greased non-stick frying pan, bake Pancetta from both sides 1-2 minutes. Remove from the fire and set aside.
2. In a meanwhile boil the eggs. To get the eggs hard-boiled, you need round 10 minutes. When done, wash the eggs with cold water well and peel off the shells.
3. In a deep bowl place ghee and add the quartered eggs. Mash with a fork well. Season it with salt and pepper to taste; add mayonnaise and mix. If you want you can pour in the Pancetta grease. Combine and mix well. Place the bowl in the fridge for one hour at least.
4. Remove the egg mixture from the fridge and make 4 equal balls.
5. Crumble the Pancetta into small pieces. Roll each ball in the Pancetta crumbles and place on a big platter.
6. Remove the Egg and Pancetta bombs in a fridge for 30 minutes more. Serve cold.

Nutrition Facts (per serving)

Total Carbohydrates: 2,2g

Dietary Fiber: 0g

Net Carbs: 0,5g

Protein: 7,5g

Total Fat: 22g

Calories: 238

Parmesan, Herb & Sun-dried Tomato Bombs

Serves 4

Ingredients

1 cup cream cheese

1 cup ghee

5 Tbsp. parmesan cheese

1/4 cup sun-dried tomatoes, chopped

1/4 cup Kalamata olives, pitted

3 cloves garlic, crushed

3 Tbsp. herbs mix (basil, parsley, thyme, oregano, parsnip, mint)

salt and freshly ground black pepper to taste

Directions

1. In a bowl, combine the cream cheese and ghee. Set aside for 30-45 minutes to soft.
2. After, mix the ghee and the cream cheese until well combined. Add the chopped Kalamata olives and sun-dried tomatoes.
3. Add in herbs and crushed garlic; season with salt and pepper to taste. Mix well with the fork and place bowl in the fridge for at least 1 hour.
4. Remove the cheese mixture from the fridge and create 4 balls. Roll each ball in the grated parmesan cheese and place on a plate.
5. Return it to the fridge for 30 minutes. Serve and enjoy.

Cooking Times

Total Time: 1 hour and 20 minutes

Nutrition Facts (per serving)

Total Carbohydrates: 4g

Dietary Fiber: 0,5g

Net Carbs: 1g

Protein: 4,6g

Total Fat: 14g

Calories: 157

Spicy Bacon & Avo Bites

Serves 6

Serving Size: 1 fat bomb

Ingredients

½ large avocado

Butter, softened (1/4 cups)

2 cloves garlic, crushed

Crushed red pepper (1 teaspoon)

½ small white onion, diced

Fresh lime juice (1 tablespoon)

Freshly ground black pepper

Sea salt (¼ teaspoon)

large slices bacon

Bacon grease, reserved from cooking (2 tablespoons)

Directions

1. Preheat the oven to 375 Fahrenheit. Line a baking tray with parchment paper. Lay the bacon strips out flat on the parchment paper, leaving space so they don't overlap. Place the tray in the oven and cook for about 10-15 minutes until golden brown and crisp. The time will depend on the thickness of the bacon slices. When done, remove from the oven and set aside to cool down.
2. Halve, deseed and peel the avocado. Place the avocado, butter, crushed red pepper, crushed garlic and lime juice into a bowl and season with salt and pepper.
3. Mash using a potato masher or a fork until well combined. Add the diced onion and mix well.

4. Pour in the 2 tablespoons of reserved bacon grease and mix well. Cover with foil and place in the fridge for 20-30 minutes to firm up.
5. Chop the bacon into small pieces and place in a shallow dish.
6. Remove the guacamole mixture from the fridge and start creating 6 balls. You can use a spoon or an ice-cream scooper. Roll each ball in the bacon crumbles and place on a tray that will fit in the fridge.
7. Eat immediately or store in the fridge in an airtight container for up to 5 days.

Nutrition Facts (per serving)

Calories: 156

Fat: 15.2

Fried Tuna & Avo Balls

Serves 12

Ingredients

Mayonnaise (1/4 cup)

Parmesan cheese (1/4 cup)

Garlic powder (1/2 teaspoon)

Salt

Canned Tuna (10 oz., drained)

Avocado (1, cubed)

Almond flour (1/3 cup)

Onion powder (1/4 teaspoon)

Coconut oil (1/2 cup)

Directions

1. Combine all ingredients in a bowl except oil and avocado.
2. Add avocado and fold, use hands to form balls and dust with flour.
3. Heat oil in a pot and fry tuna bites until golden all over.
4. Serve.

Nutritional Information per bite

Calories 135

Net Carbs 0.8g

Fats 11.8g

Protein 6.2 g

Fiber 1.2g

Bacon Zucchini Fat Bomb Balls

Ingredients

1 lb smoked bacon, crumbled

1 cup pork rinds, crushed

5 cups zucchini, minced

4 cloves garlic, minced

1 cup cream cheese

2 1/2 cup grated Parmesan cheese

4 oz goat cheese

1 tsp onion powder

1 tsp garlic powder

salt and freshly ground black pepper to taste

Directions

1. Chop or blend zucchini.
2. In large mixing bowl, combine bacon, zucchini, cream cheese, goat cheese, 1 cup grated Parmesan, minced garlic, salt and pepper to taste. Mix until all ingredients are well incorporated. Refrigerate for 2- 3 hours.
3. In a meanwhile prepare breading; in a bowl, combine crushed pork rinds, remaining 1 cup Parmesan cheese, onion powder and garlic powder.
4. Remove the zucchini mixture from the fridge and prepare about 30 even balls.
5. Roll each ball in Parmesan breading mixture until well and evenly coated. In a frying pan heat the oil.
6. Fry the zucchini bolls until they are a nice even golden brown all over. Place on a serving plate and serve hot.

Servings: 30

Cooking Times

Total Time: 20 minutes

Nutrition Facts (per serving)

Total Carbohydrates: 1,7g

Dietary Fiber: 0,25g

Net Carbs: 0,8g

Protein: 7g

Total Fat: 13g

Calories: 151

Baked Creamy Shrimps with Artichoke Hearts

Ingredients

6 oz shrimp, precooked

2 Tbsp butter

1 can (11 oz) artichoke hearts, chopped

6 scallions

1/2 cup mayonnaise

1/2 cup sour cream

1 cup Cheddar cheese, shredded

1 1/4 cup Parmesan cheese, shredded

1 Tbsp garlic, minced

1 tsp red pepper flakes

1 tsp garlic powder

Directions

1. Preheat oven to 350F.
2. In a frying pan, sauté shrimps over medium heat with butter and red pepper flakes for 5-10 minutes. Chop the artichoke hearts.
3. In a bowl, combine all your ingredient and mix until well blended.
4. Pour the mixture in a baking dish and bake for 30 minutes in preheated oven. Serve hot.

Servings: 16

Cooking Times

Total Time: 40 minutes

Nutrition Facts (per serving)

Total Carbohydrates: 6,32g

Dietary Fiber: 1,6g

Net Carbs: 1g

Protein: 8g

Total Fat: 11g

Calories: 150

Blue Cheese Turkey Dressed Eggs

Ingredients

6 eggs

2 green onions

6 oz smoked turkey breast, chopped

1/2 cup blue cheese, crumbled

2 Tbsp Blue cheese dressing

1/4 cup mayonnaise

2 Tbsp hot mustard

1/2 rib celery

Directions

1. Hard boil the eggs, covered for 12 minutes.
2. In a meanwhile, chop up the smoked turkey breast and the celery.
3. Slice eggs in half lengthwise, scrape the yolks out into a bowl. Add the rest of the ingredients (except the green onions).
4. Grate the green onions over the mixture. Mix all ingredients together.
5. With the teaspoon fill every egg with the mixture.
6. Place on a serving plate and refrigerate for one hour. Ready! Serve and enjoy!

Servings: 6

Cooking Times

Total Time: 20 minutes

Nutrition Facts (per serving)

Total Carbohydrates: 3,9g

Dietary Fiber: 0,3g

Net Carbs: 0,6g

Protein: 14g

Total Fat: 11,5g

Calories: 167

Olives and Sun-dried Tomatoes Fat Bombs

Ingredients

1 cup cream cheese

1 cup ghee

5 Tbsp parmesan cheese

1/4 cup sun-dried tomatoes, chopped

1/4 cup Kalamata olives, pitted

3 cloves garlic, crushed

3 Tbsp herbs mix (basil, parsley, thyme, oregano, parsnip, mint)

salt and freshly ground black pepper to taste

Directions

1. In a bowl, combine the cream cheese and ghee. Set aside for 30-45 minutes to soft.
2. After, mix the ghee and the cream cheese until well combined. Add the chopped Kalamata olives and sun-dried tomatoes.
3. Add in herbs and crushed garlic; season with salt and pepper to taste. Mix well with the fork and place bowl in the fridge for at least 1 hour.
4. Remove the cheese mixture from the fridge and create 4 balls. Roll each ball in the grated parmesan cheese and place on a plate.
5. Return it to the fridge for 30 minutes. Serve and enjoy.

Servings: 4

Cooking Times

Total Time: 1 hour and 20 minutes

Nutrition Facts (per serving)

Total Carbohydrates: 4g

Dietary Fiber: 0,5g

Net Carbs: 1g

Protein: 4,6g

Total Fat: 14g

Calories: 157

Pork Ham, Sausages and Cashews Truffles

Ingredients

8 slices smoked pork ham

8 oz sausages

6 oz cream cheese, softened

1 cup cashews, chopped

1 tsp Dijon mustard

Directions

1. In a food processor blend chopped sausages and cashews.
2. In a separate bowl, beat the cream cheese and mustard until soft.
3. Roll the sausage mixture into 12 small balls. Take each ball and form layer of cream cheese with your fingers.
4. Refrigerate for about 45-60 minutes.
5. Roll each ball in the finely chopped smoked pork ham and place on a serving dish. Serve.

Servings: 12

Total Time: 15 minutes

Nutrition Facts (per serving)

Total Carbohydrates: 1,5g

Net Carbs: 0,5g

Protein: 7g

Total Fat: 11g

Calories: 125

Smoked Mackerel Fat Bombs

Ingredients

2 oz smoked mackerel fish

2.7 oz butter, grass-fed

3.5 oz cream cheese

1 Tbsp fresh lemon juice

pinch of salt

Directions

1. In a food processor put butter, cream cheese, smoked mackerel fish and fresh lemon juice. Blend until all ingredients incorporate well.
2. Line a tray with parchment paper and create 6 fat bombs. Place in the fridge for 2 hours or until firm. Serve.

Servings: 6

Cooking Time: 5 minutes

Nutrition Facts (per serving)

Total Carbohydrates: 0,8g

Net Carbs: 0,6g

Protein: 3,3g

Total Fat: 17g

Calories: 163

Bacon Fat Bomb Dip

Ingredients

6 slices bacon, cooked and crumbled

2 cups sour cream

1 cup cream cheese

1 1 cups Cheddar cheese, shredded

1 cup sliced scallions, white and green parts

Directions

1. Preheat oven to 400 F
2. In a deep bowl, combine all ingredients. Spoon mixture into a baking dish and bake until cheese is bubbling, about 25-30 minutes.
3. Once ready, let cool and serve hot.

Servings: 18

Cooking Time: 35 minutes

Nutrition Facts (per serving)

Total Carbohydrates: 1,7g

Net Carbs: 1,4g

Protein: 5,5g

Total Fat: 19g

Calories: 197

Turkey Bacon and Avocado Stuffed Eggs

Ingredients

6 eggs

1 avocado

6 slices smoked turkey bacon

2 Tbsp mustard

1 Tbsp garlic, minced

1 Tbsp lime juice

1 Tbsp dried onion flakes

pinch Cayenne pepper, or to taste

1 tsp garlic salt

Directions

1. Hard boil the eggs (about 12 minutes). Peel the eggs and slice in half lengthwise
2. In a large mixing bowl mash the avocado.
3. Scrape the yolks out into the mixing bowl. Add in the bacon, mustard, cayenne pepper, lime juice, onion flakes, garlic and garlic salt. Mix it well until smooth and creamy.
4. Fill every egg half with the avocado mixture. Refrigerate stuffed eggs for one hour. Serve.

Servings: 6

Cooking Times

Total Time: 30 minutes

Nutrition Facts (per serving)

Total Carbohydrates: 4,4g

Dietary Fiber: 2,3g

Net Carbs: 0,5g

Protein: 9g

Total Fat: 13g

Calories: 162

Protein 9,36g 19%

Hot Hot Fat Bombs

Ingredients

1/2 cup Cream cheese

4 slices Pepperoni Sausages (or any salami made from cured pork and beef mixed together)

3 slices smoked bacon

1 medium Chili pepper

1/2 tsp dried basil

1/4 tsp onion powder

1/4 tsp garlic powder

salt and pepper to taste

Directions

1. In a frying pan brown 3 slices of bacon and Peperoni sausages until crisp.
2. Remove bacon and Pepperoni from the pan on a paper lined plate to cool. Keep the remaining grease for later use.
3. Dice Chilli pepper into small pieces.
4. Combine cream cheese, chilli pepper and spices. Add the bacon fat in and mix together until a solid mixture is formed. Season with salt and pepper to taste.
5. Crumble bacon and Pepperone slices and set on a plate. Roll cream cheese mixture into balls using your hand, then roll the ball into the bacon or Pepperone.

Servings: 6

Cooking Times

Total Time: 15 minutes

Nutrition Facts (per serving)

Total Carbohydrates: 1,3g

Dietary Fiber: 0,11g

Net Carbs: 0,6g

Protein: 4g

Total Fat: 16g

Calories: 165

Wrapped Bacon Rolls

Ingredients

4 bacon slice

6 toasted pecan halves, chopped

1/2 cup unsalted butter

1/2 cup of Mayonnaise

granulated garlic (to taste)

Directions

1. Divide bacon into 3 equal parts.
2. Spread generously each bacon part with unsalted butter. Press butter side into pecan pieces.
3. Top with each with a mayonnaise, sprinkle with granulated garlic and wrap in a rolls. Enjoy!!

Servings: 12

Cooking Time: 10 minutes

Nutrition Facts (per serving)

Total Carbohydrates: 2,7g

Dietary Fiber: 0,15g

Net Carbs: 0,7g

Protein: 1,78g

Total Fat: 17,7g

Calories: 174

Lettuce with Prosciutto and Butternut Squash

Ingredients

3 strips Prosciutto

1 cup butternut squash, cubed

1/4 cup sour cream

3 Tbsp thinly sliced fresh chives

6 lettuce leaves

Kosher salt and freshly ground black pepper

Directions

1. In a frying pan, cook the bacon about 3 minutes. Add the butternut squash and salt and pepper to taste. Cook, stirring 6 - 8 minutes. Add in the chives and adjust salt and pepper to taste. Let cool for several minutes.
2. Chop the bacon and add all other ingredients (except lettuce) and mix well.
3. Set the lettuce leaves on a large platter. Top each leave with a dollop of the bacon-sour cream-butternut squash mixture and then sprinkle with some chopped chives. Serve immediately.

Servings: 6

Cooking Time: 35 minutes

Nutrition Facts (per serving)

Total Carbohydrates: 4g

Net Carbs: 1,05g

Protein: 2,76g

Total Fat: 11g

Calories: 120

Pancetta Wrapped Provolone Sticks

Ingredients

4 slices Pancetta bacon

2 Frigo string Provolone cheese (or Mozzarela, Kasseri, Emmenthal...)

1/2 cup coconut oil for frying

toothpicks

Directions

1. Preheat your coconut oil in a deep fryer to 350 degrees.
2. Wrap your cut in half Provolone cheese sticks with the Pancetta. At the end of the wrapping, secure with a toothpick.
3. Drop the bacon wrapped cheese in the hot oil and cook about 2-3 minutes, depending on the thickness of your bacon.
4. Remove your Pancetta Wrapped Provolone Sticks to a paper towel to cool for a few minutes. Remove the toothpick and serve.

Servings: 10

Nutrition Facts (per serving)

Total Carbohydrates: 0,42g

Dietary Fiber: 0g

Net Carbs: 0,08g

Protein: 5,6g

Total Fat: 22g

Calories: 216

Savory Coco Bacon Bombs

Ingredients

8 strips cooked crispy bacon, crumbled

1 cup cream cheese, softened

1/2 cup butter

4 tsp bacon fat

4 Tbsp coconut oil

1/4 cup Splenda to taste

Directions

1. In a microwave dish, combine all ingredients and melt slowly in the microwave until smooth. Set aside some crumbled bacon,
2. Pour into a dish or pan and place in the freezer until firm, about 30 minutes.
3. Before serving, remove from freezer, sprinkle with more crumbled bacon, slice and serve.

Servings: 24

Nutrition Facts (per serving)

Total Carbohydrates: 0,5g

Dietary Fiber: 0g

Net Carbs: 0,3g

Protein: 0g

Total Fat: 15,9g

Calories: 151

Scrambled Eggs Muffins

Ingredients

3 strips of crumbled cooked bacon

6 six eggs

2 Tbsp Coconut oil or butter

1 Tbsp butter

1/4 cup softened cream cheese

1/4 cup shredded Gouda cheese

garlic & onion powder

black or white pepper

Directions

1. In small bowl, melt the butter and set aside. In a separate bowl beat the eggs. Add in spices.Heat some butter in a non stick skille on medium heat and scramble the eggs .
2. Put cooked eggs into another large bowl. Put in your cheeses and mix well. Add bacon and stir. Add the melted butter and coconut oil.
3. Pour the batter in mini muffin liners. Place on cookie sheet with or without wax paper, and freeze for about 30 minutes. Serve.

Servings: 8

Cooking Times

Total Time: 15 minutes

Nutrition Facts (per serving)

Total Carbohydrates: 0,54g

Dietary Fiber: 0g

Net Carbs: 0,3g

Protein: 7,9g

Total Fat: 16,9g

Calories: 186

Sugar 0,31g

Smoked Salmon Cream Cheese Balls

Ingredients

2 oz smoked salmon fillets

1/2 cup cream cheese

3 oz butter, grass-fed

1 Tbs fresh lemon juice

pinch salt

Directions

1. In a food processor put butter, cream cheese, smoked mackere and fresh lemon juice. Blend until all ingredients incorporate well.
2. Line a tray with parchment paper and create 6 Balls. Place in the fridge for 2 hours or until firm.
3. Serve.

Servings: 6

Cooking Time: 5 minutes

Nutrition Facts (per serving)

Total Carbohydrates: 0,87g

Dietary Fiber: 0.1g

Net Carbs: 0,6g

Protein: 3,29g

Total Fat: 16,62g

Calories: 163,41

Breading Kohlrabi & Bacon Rind

Ingredients

1 lb smoked bacon, crumbled

5 cups kohlrabi, minced

1 cup pork rinds, crushed

2 1/2 cup grated Parmesan cheese

4 oz mascarpone cheese

4 cloves garlic, minced

1 cup cream cheese

1 tsp onion powder

1 tsp garlic powder

salt ad freshly ground black pepper to taste

Directions

1. Chop or blend kohlrabi.
2. In large mixing bowl, combine kohlrabi, bacon, cream cheese, mascarpone cheese, 1 cup grated Parmesan, minced garlic, salt and pepper to taste. Mix until all ingredients are well incorporated. Refrigerate for 2- 3 hours.
3. For breading: In a bowl, combine crushed pork rinds, remaining 1 cup Parmesan cheese, onion powder and garlic powder.
4. Remove the kohlrabi mixture from the fridge and prepare about 30 even balls.
5. In a frying pan heat the oil. Roll each ball in Parmesan breading mixture until well and evenly coated. Fry the kohlrabi balls until they are a nice even golden brown all over. Place on a serving plate and serve hot.

Servings: 30

Cooking Times

Total Time: 20 minutes

Nutrition Facts (per serving)

Total Carbohydrates: 2,5g

Dietary Fiber: 0,9g

Net Carbs: 1g

Protein: 7,5g

Total Fat: 13g

Calories: 154

Dessert Recipes

Pecan Blondie's

Serves 16

Ingredients

3 eggs

2 1/4 cups pecans, roasted

3 Tbs heavy cream

1 Tbs salted caramel syrup

1/2 cup flax seeds, ground

1/4 cup butter, melted

1/4 cup erythritol, powdered

10 drops Liquid Stevia

1 tsp baking powder

1 pinch salt

Directions

1. Preheat oven to 350F.
2. In a baking pan roast pecans for 10 minutes.
3. Grind 1/2 cup flax seeds in a spice grinder. Place flax seed powder in a bowl. Grind Erythritol in a spice grinder until powdered. Set in the same bowl as the flax seeds meal.
4. Place 2/3 of roasted pecans in food processor and process until a smooth nut butter is formed.
5. Add eggs, liquid Stevia, salted caramel syrup, and a pinch of salt to the flax seed mixture. Mix well. Add pecan butter to the batter and mix again.

6. Smash the rest of the roasted pecans into chunks. Add crushed pecans and 1/4 cup melted butter into the batter.
7. Mix batter well, and then add heavy cream and baking powder. Mix everything together well.
8. Place the batter into baking tray and bake for 20 minute. Let cool for about 10 minutes. Slice off the edges of the brownie to create a uniform square. Serve.

Cooking Time: 40 minutes

Amount Per Serving

Total Carbs 3,54g

Calories 180,45

Total Fat 18,23g

Fiber 1,78g

Sugar 1,45g

Protein 3,07g

Chocolate Minty Ice Cream

Serves 3

Ingredients

1/2 tsp Peppermint extract

1 cup heavy cream

1 cup cheese cream

1 tsp pure vanilla extract

1 tsp Liquid Stevia extract

100% Dark Chocolate for topping

Directions

1. Place ice cream bowl in freezer per ice cream maker instructions. In a metal bowl, put all ingredients except chocolate and whisk well.
2. Put back in freezer for 5 minutes. Setup ice cream maker and add liquid.
3. Before serving, top the ice cream with chocolate shavings. Serve.

Cooking Time: 35 minutes

Amount Per Serving

Total Carbs 2,7g

Calories 286,66

Total Fat 29,96g

Sugar 0,9g

Protein 2,6g

Coconut Waffles

Serves 8

Ingredients

1 cup coconut flour

1/2 cup heavy (whipping) cream

5 eggs

1/4 tsp pink salt

1/4 tsp baking soda

1/4 cup coconut milk

2 tsp Yacon Syrup (or some other natural sweetener)

2 Tbsp coconut oil (melted)

Directions

1. In a large bowl add the eggs and beat with an electric hand mixer for 30 seconds.
2. Add the heavy (whipping) cream and coconut oil into the eggs while you are still mixing. Add the coconut milk, coconut flour, pink salt and baking soda. Mix with the hand mixer for 45 second on low speed. Set aside.
3. Heat up your waffle maker well and make the waffles according to your manufactures specifications.
4. Serve hot.

Amount Per Serving

Calories 169,21

Total Fat 12,6g 19%

Total Carbs 9,97g 3%

Fiber 0,45g 2%

Sugar 0,38g

Protein 4,39g 9%

Choc- Raspberry Cream

Serves 4

Ingredients

1/2 cup 100% dark chocolate, chopped

1/4 cup of heavy cream

1/2 cup cream cheese, softened

2 Tbsp sugar free Raspberry Syrup

1/4 cup Erythritol

Directions

1. In a double boiler melt chopped chocolate and the cream cheese. Add the Erythritol sweetener and continue to stir. Remove from heat, let cool and set aside.
2. When the cream has cooled add in heavy cream and Raspberry syrup and stir well.
3. Pour cream in a bowls or glasses and serve. Keep refrigerated.

Cooking Time: 15 minutes

Amount Per Serving

Total Carbs 7,47g 2%

Calories 157,67

Total Fat 13,51g 21%

Fiber 1g 4%

Sugar 5,16g

Protein 1,95g 4%

Hazelnut & Cacao Cookies

Serves 24

Ingredients

2 cups almond flour

1 cup chopped hazelnut

1/2 cup cacao powder

1/2 cup ground flax

3 Tbsp coconut oil (melted)

1/3 cup water

1/3 cup Erythritol

1/4 tsp liquid Stevia

Directions

1. In a bowl, mix almond flour and flax and cacao powder. Stir in oil, water, agave and vanilla. When it is well mixed, stir in chopped hazelnuts.
2. Form in to balls, press flat with palms and place on dehydrator screens.
3. Dehydrate 1 hour at 145, then reduce to 116 and dehydrate for at least 5 hours or until desired dryness is achieved.
4. Serve.

Cooking Time: 6 hours

Amount Per Serving

Total Carbs 8,75g

Calories 181,12

Total Fat 15,69g

Fiber 3,45g

Sugar 3,75g

Protein 4,46g

Dark Chocolate Brownies

Serves 16

Ingredients

3 eggs

4 oz dark chocolate, unsweetened

1/2 cup coconut oil

1 cup almond flour

1 cup walnuts

2 Tbs cocoa, unsweetened

1 tsp vanilla essence

2 cups granulated sweetener Stevia or Erythritol

1 tsp baking soda

pinch of salt

Directions

1. Preheat the oven to 350F.
2. In a container, add almond flour, sweetener, cocoa, salt and baking soda. With an electric mixer, blend the ingredients on the slowest setting until combined well.
3. Melt the chocolate and the coconut oil together (In a microwave or double boiler). Stir thoroughly.
4. Add eggs and vanilla essence to the flour and mix on a medium speed until a thick batter is formed.
5. Add the butter/chocolate mix to the batter continuing on medium speed until an even texture is formed. Line a slice tin or square baking tin with wax paper. Fold in walnut pieces then turn the batter into your slice tin.
6. Bake for 25 minutes. When ready let cool on wire rack.

7. Cut into 16 Brownies and serve.

Cooking Times

Total Time: 35 minutes

Amount Per Serving

Total Carbs 5,38g

Calories 207,88

Total Fat 20,72g

Fiber 2,82g

Sugar 0,73g

Protein 5,14g

Rich Almond Butter Cake & Chocolate Sauce

Serves 12

Ingredients

1 cup almond butter or soaked almonds

1/4 cup almond milk, unsweetened

1 cup coconut oil

2 tsp liquid Stevia sweetener to taste

Topping: Chocolate Sauce

4 Tbsp cocoa powder, unsweetened

2 Tbsp almond butter

2 Tbsp Stevia sweetener

Directions

1. Melt the coconut oil in room temperature.
2. Add all ingredients in a bowl and blend well until combined.
3. Pour the almond butter mixture into a parchment lined platter.
4. Place in refrigerator for 3 hours.
5. In a bowl, whisk all topping ingredients together. Pour over the almond cake after it's been set. Cut into cubes and serve.

Cooking Time: 5 minutes

Nutrition Facts (per serving)

Total Carbohydrates: 9,8g

Dietary Fiber: 2g

Net Carbs:2,4g

Protein: 5,8g

Total Fat: 23,3g

Calories: 273

Peanut Butter Cake Covered in Chocolate Sauce

Serves 12

Ingredients

1 cup peanut butter

1/4 cup almond milk, unsweetened

1 cup coconut oil

2 tsp liquid Stevia sweetener to taste

Topping: Chocolate Sauce

2 Tbsp coconut oil, melted

4 Tbsp cocoa powder, unsweetened

2 Tbsp Stevia sweetener

Directions

1. In a microwave bowl mix coconut oil and peanut butter; melt in a microwave for 1-2 minutes.
2. Add this mixture to your blender; add in the rest of the ingredients and blend well until combined.
3. Pour the peanut mixture into a parchment lined loaf pan or platter.
4. Refrigerate for about 3 hours; the longer, the better.
5. In a bowl, whisk all topping ingredients together. Pour over the peanut candy after it's been set. Cut into cubes and serve.

Cooking Time: 5 minutes

Nutrition Facts (per serving)

Total Carbohydrates: 5,8g

Dietary Fiber: 2g

Net Carbs: 2,4g

Protein: 6g

Total Fat: 27g

Calories: 273

Spicy Pumpkin Ice Cream

Serves 6

Ingredients

1 cup almond milk (unsweetened)

1 cup coconut milk

1 cup pumpkin puree

2 1/2 tsp ground cinnamon

1 tsp pure vanilla extract

1/2 tsp ground ginger

1/2 tsp nutmeg

1/8 tsp sea salt

Thickener:

1/2 tsp guar gum or 1 tablespoon gelatin dissolved in 1/4 cup boiling water

Directions

1. Put the coconut milk in a blender and purée until smooth.
2. Pour into the ice cream machine or blender and churn well. Serve in chilled glasses.
3. Freeze for about an hour or refrigerate until cold.
4. Add the almond milk, pumpkin puree, vanilla, cinnamon, ginger, nutmeg and salt, plus thickener. Purée until smooth.
5. Serve.

Cooking Times

Inactive Time: 1 hour

Total Time: 15 minutes

Nutrition Facts (per serving)

Total Carbs 4,73g

Calories 118,25

Total Fat 11,3g

Fiber 1,4g 6%

Sugar 1,43g

Protein 1,35g

All-stars Peanut-Butter Cookies

Ingredients

2 cups peanut butter

1/4 cup Erythritol

2 eggs

1 1/4 cups coconut flour

2 tsp baking soda

2 tsp peanut extract

1/2 tsp kosher salt

Directions

1. Preheat oven to 345° F.
2. In a bowl beat the peanut butter, coconut flour and Erythritol with an electric mixer (MEDIUM speed) until fluffy. Reduce speed to LOW and add in the eggs, baking soda, vanilla, and salt.
3. With your hands make balls from the batter and place on parchment-lined baking pan. Bake 10 to 15 minutes. When ready, cool slightly and then move from the stove to cool completely. Ready. Serve.

Servings: 18

Cooking Times

Total Time: 1 hour and 15 minutes

Nutrition Facts (per serving)

Calories 182,5

Total Fat 14,67g 23%

Total Carbohydrates 8,65g 3%

Fiber 1,96g 8%

Protein 7g 14%

Chocolate Almond Brownies

Ingredients

3 eggs

4 oz dark chocolate, unsweetened

1/2 cup coconut oil

1 cup almond flour

1 cup walnuts

2 Tbs cocoa, unsweetened

1 tsp vanilla essence

2 cups granulated sweetener Stevia or Erythritol

1 tsp baking soda

pinch of salt

Directions

1. Preheat the oven to 350F.
2. In a container, add almond flour, sweetener, cocoa, salt and baking soda. With an electric mixer, blend the ingredients on the slowest setting until combined well.
3. Melt the chocolate and the coconut oil together (In a microwave or double boiler). Stir thoroughly.
4. Add eggs and vanilla essence to the flour and mix on a medium speed until a thick batter is formed.
5. Add the butter/chocolate mix to the batter continuing on medium speed until an even texture is formed. Line a slice tin or square baking tin with wax paper. Fold in walnut pieces then turn the batter into your slice tin.
6. Bake for 25 minutes. When ready let cool on wire rack.
7. Cut into 16 Brownies and serve.

Servings: 16

Cooking Times

Total Time: 35 minutes

Nutrition Facts (per serving)

Calories 207,88

Total Fat 20,72g 32%

Total Carbohydrates 5,38g 2%

Fiber 2,82g 11%

Protein 5,14g 10%

Almond Choc Cookies

Ingredients

2 cups almond meal

1 1/2 tsp almond extract

4 Tbsp cocoa powder

5 Tbsp coconut oil, melted

2 Tbsp almond milk

4 Tbsp agave nectar

2 tsp vanilla extract

1/8 tsp baking soda

1/8 tsp salt

Directions

1. Preheat oven to 340F degrees.
2. In a deep bowl mix salt, cocoa powder, almond meal and baking soda.
3. In a separate bowl, whisk together melted coconut oil, almond milk, almond and vanilla extract and maple syrup. Merge the almond meal mixture with almond milk mixture and mix well.
4. In a greased baking pan pour the batter evenly. Bake for 10-15 minutes. 5. Once ready let cool on a wire rack and serve.

Servings: 12

Cooking Times

Total Time: 25 minutes

Nutrition Facts (per serving)

Calories 79,32

Total Fat 5,94g 9%

Total Carbohydrates 7,02g 2%

Fiber 0,61g 2%

Protein 0,46g <1%

Carrot Flowers Muffins

Ingredients

2 eggs

2 cups shredded carrots

1/4 cup coconut flour

1/2 cup coconut oil

1 tsp vanilla extract

1/4 cup Erythritol

2 tsp ground cinnamon

1 tsp baking powder

Directions

1. Preheat oven to 350F. Prepare12 muffin tins.
2. In your food processor, add in carrots, eggs, coconut oil, Erythritol, and vanilla. Blend together until combined.
3. In a separate bowl, mix together coconut flour, cinnamon and baking powder.
4. Pour the carrot mixture into the dry ingredients and mix until completely combined.
5. Pour carrot mixture into the muffin tin and bake for about 30-35 minutes.
6. Remove from the oven, and let cool for at least 30 minutes. Serve.

Servings: 12

Cooking Times

Total Time: 50 minutes

Nutrition Facts (per serving)

Calories 127,55

Total Fat 10,04g 15%

Total Carbohydrates 8,81g 3%

Fiber 0,91g 4%

Protein 1,53g 3%

Coconut Jelly Cake

Ingredients

1 cup coconut flour

1/2 cup butter, softened

2 Tbs raspberry jelly

1/2 cup coconut sugar

3 cups desiccated coconut

1 egg

2/3 cup coconut milk

1 cup boiling water

1 cup cold water

1/2 cup double thick cream

Directions

1. Preheat oven to 360F. Grease a patty pan.
2. In a bowl beat butter and coconut sugar until light. Add in egg and beat until well combined. Gently fold in half the coconut flour and half the milk. Repeat with remaining flour and milk.
3. Spoon mixture into patty pan. Bake for 15 to 20 minutes. Once ready, let cool cakes on a wire rack.
4. Stir jelly and boiling water together in a bowl until crystals are dissolved. Stir in cold water. Refrigerate for 1 hour.
5. Place coconut into a large bowl. Cut each cake in half. Stick halves back together using 1 teaspoon of cream. Using a slotted spoon lower cakes, 1 cake at a time, into jelly. Drain excess jelly.
1. 6.Toss cakes in coconut until well coated. When ready, place onto a lined tray and refrigerate at least 1 hour or until set.

Servings: 18

Cooking Times

Total Time: 30 minutes

Nutrition Facts (per serving)

Calories 146,51

Total Fat 14,31g 22%

Total Carbohydrates 4,21g 1%

Fiber 2,16g 9%

Protein 1,83g 4%

Cottage Pumpkin Pie Ice Cream

Ingredients

1/2 cup toasted pecans, chopped

3 egg yolks

2 Tbsp butter, salted

2 cups coconut milk

1/2 cup pumpkin puree

1 tsp pumpkin spice

1/2 cup cottage cheese

1/2 tsp chia seeds

1/3 cup Erythritol

20 drops liquid Nutria

Directions

1. Place all ingredients into a container of your immersion blender. Blend all of the ingredients together into a smooth mixture.
2. Add mixture to your ice cream machine, as per instructions of your manufacturer.
3. Follow the churning instructions as per your ice cream maker manufacturer's instructions. Serve in a chilled bowls or glasses.

Servings: 6

Cooking Times

Total Time: 15 minutes

Nutrition Facts (per serving)

Calories 233,69

Total Fat 21,74g 33%

Total Carbohydrates 6,87g 2%

Fiber 1,95g 8%

Protein 5,49g 11%

Divine Chocolate Biscotti

Ingredients

1 egg

2 cups whole almonds

2 Tbs flax seeds

1 cup shredded coconut, unsweetened

1 cup coconut oil

1 cup cacao powder

1/4 cup Xilitol or Stevia sweetener

1 tsp salt

1 tsp baking soda

Directions

1. Preheat oven to 350F.
2. In a food process blend the whole almonds with the flax seeds. Add in the rest of ingredients and mix well.
3. Place the dough on a piece of aluminum foil to shape into 8 biscotti-shaped slices. Bake for 12 minutes.
4. Let cool and serve.

Servings: 8

Cooking Times

Total Time: 25 minutes

Nutrition Facts (per serving)

Calories 276,56

Total Fat 25,44g 39%

Total Carbohydrates 9,19g 3%

Fiber 5,2g 21%

Protein 8,24g 16%

Hemp and Chia Seeds Cream

Ingredients

1 ¼ cup coconut milk

2 Tbsp hemp powder

2 sheets of unflavored gelatin

3 Tbsp chia seeds

Directions

1. In a saucepan over low heat add the coconut milk and dissolve the lucuma powder.
2. Cut the gelatin into pieces and add it to the milk. Stir until dissolved completely.
3. Add chia seeds and stir occasionally until mixture thickens, about 15 minutes. Pour the mixture into individual containers and allow cool before putting them in the refrigerator for at least 2 hours before serving. Enjoy!

Servings: 3

Cooking Time: 20 minutes

Nutrition Facts (per serving)

Calories 202,43

Total Fat 19,2g 30%

Total Carbohydrates 8,12g 3%

Fiber 3,14g 13%

Protein 2,59g 5%

Homemade Nuts Bars

Ingredients

1 cup almonds

1/2 cup hazelnut, chopped

1 cup peanuts

1 cup shredded coconut

1 cup almond butter

1 cup Liquid Erythritol

1 cup coconut oil, freshly melted and still warm

Directions

1. In a food processor place all nuts and chop for 1-2 minutes.
2. Add in grated coconut, almond butter, Erythritol and coconut oil. Process it for 1 minute about.
3. Cover a square bowl with parchment paper and place the mixture on top.
4. Flatten the mixture with a spatula. Place the bowl in the freezer for 4-5 hours.
5. Remove batter from the freezer, cut and serve.

Servings: 10

Cooking Times

Cooking Time: 10 minutes

Inactive Time: 5 hours

Nutrition Facts (per serving)

Calories 193,62

Total Fat 18,2g 28%

Total Carbohydrates 6,64g 2%

Fiber 2,53g 10%

Protein 3,83g 8%

Caramel Coffee Smoothie

Ingredients

1/2 cup heavy cream

1/2 cup almond milk, unsweetened

3 Tbsp sugar-free chocolate syrup

3 Tbsp sugar-free caramel syrup

3/4 cup cold coffee

2 Tbs cocoa, unsweetened

Ice cubes

Directions

1. In a blender add all ingredients and blend until all incorporate well.
2. Pour in glasses and serve.

Servings: 4

Cooking Times

Total Time: 5 minutes

Nutrition Facts (per serving)

Calories 170,62

Total Fat 14,95g 23%

Total Carbohydrates 9,02g 3%

Fiber 1,92g 8%

Protein 2,8g 6%

Chocolate Chia Cream

Ingredients

1/4 cup Chia seeds

1 cup heavy whipping cream

1 cup coconut milk

2 Tbs cocoa powder

pure vanilla extract

1/4 cup Erythritol sweetener

Directions

1. In a bowl mix the chia seeds and add the coconut milk until it combines well.
2. Add the Erythritol and whisk some more. Divide the mixture into two portions.
3. Add cocoa to one half and mixed it nicely.
4. Pour chia seed mixture into the bowls or glasses. Keep covered in the refrigerator for 12 hours.
1. Before serving beat the heavy whipping cream and pour over the chia seeds cream. Enjoy!

Servings: 4

Cooking Times

Total Time: 12 hours

Nutrition Facts (per serving)

Calories 341,31

Total Fat 35,41g 54%

Total Carbohydrates 7,35g 2%

Fiber 1,56g 6%

Protein 2,99g 6%

Chocolate Brownies

Ingredients

2 eggs

1 1/2 cups almond flour

1/4 cup coconut oil

1/2 cup cocoa powder, unsweetened

1 Tbs Metamucil Fiber Powder

1/3 cup Natvia (or some other natural sweetener)l

1/4 cup maple syrup

1 tsp baking powder

1/2 tsp salt

Directions

1. Preheat oven to 350F.
2. In a bowl add in all wet ingredients and 2 Eggs. Beat the wet ingredients together using a hand mixer until a consistent mixture is formed.
3. In a separate bowl, combine all dry ingredients. Mix the dry ingredients well. Pour the wet ingredients slowly into the dry ingredients, mixing with a hand mixer as you pour.
4. Pour the batter into baking pan. Bake the brownies for 20 minutes.
5. When ready, let the brownies cool. Slice brownies into slices and serve.

Servings: 10

Cooking Times

Total Time: 35 minutes

Nutrition Facts (per serving)

Calories 157,81

Total Fat 13,4g 21%

Total Carbohydrates 8,07g 3%

Fiber 2,58g 10%

Protein 5,04g 10%

Chocolate Pecan Bites

Ingredients

2 oz 100% dark chocolate

2.5 oz pecan halves

cinnamon

nutmeg

Directions

1. Preheat oven to 350F.
2. Place the pecan halves on a parchment paper and bake in oven for 6-7 minutes. When ready, let cool and set aside.
3. Melt the dark chocolate.
4. Dip each pecan half in the melted dark chocolate and place back on the parchment paper.
5. Sprinkle a cinnamon and nutmeg on top of the chocolate covered pecans.
6. Before serving place in refrigerator for 2-3 hours.

Servings: 12

Cooking Time: 3 hours

Nutrition Facts (per serving)

Calories 52,13

Total Fat 4,96g 8%

Total Carbohydrates 2,32g <1%

Fiber 0,71g 3%

Protein 0,64g 1%

Hazelnuts Chocolate Cream

Ingredients

1 cup hazelnuts halves

4 Tbsp unsweetened cocoa powder

1 tsp pure vanilla extract

2 Tbsp coconut oil

4 Tbsp granulated Stevia (or sweetener of choice)

Directions

1. Place all the ingredients in your blender. Blend until smooth well.
2. Store in the fridge for 1 hour. Serve and enjoy!

Servings: 4

Cooking Times

Total Time: 5 minutes

Nutrition Facts (per serving)

Calories 302,88

Total Fat 29,65g 46%

Total Carbohydrates 9,5g 3%

Fiber 5,12g 20%

Protein 6,39g 13%

Instant Coffee Ice Cream

Ingredients

1 Tbsp Instant Coffee

2 Tbsp Cocoa Powder

1 cup coconut milk

1/4 cup heavy cream

1/4 tsp flax seeds

2 Tbs Erythritol

15 drops liquid Nutria

Directions

1. Add all ingredients except the flax seeds into a container of your immersion blender.
2. Blend well until all ingredients are incorporated well. Slowly add in flax seeds until a slightly thicker mixture is formed. Add the mass to your ice cream machine and follow manufacturer's instructions.
3. Ready! Serve!

Servings: 2

Cooking Times

Total Time: 20 minutes

Nutrition Facts (per serving)

Calories 286,99

Total Fat 29,21g 45%

Total Carbohydrates 9,39g 3%

Fiber 1,88g 8%

Protein 3,18g 6%

Jam "Eye" Cookies

Ingredients

2 eggs

1 cup almond flour

2 Tbsp coconut flour

2 Tbsp sugar-free jam per taste

1/2 cup natural sweetener (Stevia, Truvia, Erythritol...etc.)

4 Tbs coconut oil

1/2 tsp pure vanilla extract

1/2 tsp almond extract

1 Tbs shredded coconut

1/2 tsp baking powder

1/4 tsp cinnamon

1/2 tsp salt

Directions

1. Preheat your oven to 350F. In a big bowl, combine all your dry ingredients and whisk.
2. Add in your wet ingredients and combine well using hand mixer or a whisk.
3. With your hand for make the patties and place the cookies on a parchment paper lined baking sheet. Using your finger make an indent in the middle if each cookie.
4. Bake for about 16 minutes or until the cookies turn golden.
5. Once ready, let the cookies cool on a wire rack and fill each indent with sugar free jam.
6. Before serving sprinkle some shredded coconut on top of each cookie. Enjoy!

Servings: 16

Cooking Times

Total Time: 36 minutes

Nutrition Facts (per serving)

Calories 95,1

Total Fat 8,61g 13%

Total Carbohydrates 2,79g <1%

Fiber 1,02g 4%

Protein 2,71g 5%

Lemon Coconut Pearls

Ingredients

3 packages of True Lemon (Crystallized Citrus for Water)

1/4 cup shredded coconut, unsweetened

1 cup cream cheese

1/4 cup granulated Stevia

Directions

1. In a bowl, combine cream cheese, lemon and Stevia. Blend well until incorporate.
2. Once the mixture is well combined, put it back in the fridge to harden up a bit.
3. Roll into 16 balls and dip each ball into shredded coconut. Refrigerate for several hours. Serve.

Servings: 4

Cooking Time: 15 minutes

Nutrition Facts (per serving)

Calories 216,06

Total Fat 21,53g 33%

Total Carbohydrates 3,12g 1%

Fiber 0,45g 2%

Protein 3,61g 7%

Lime & Vanilla Cheesecake

Ingredients

1/4 cup cream cheese, softened

2 Tbsp heavy cream

1 tsp lime juice

1 egg

1 tsp pure vanilla extract

2-4 Tbsp Eerythritol or Stevia

Directions

1. In a microwave-safe bowl combine all ingredients. Place in a microwave and cook on HIGH for 90 seconds.
2. Every 30 seconds stir to combine the ingredients well.
3. Transfer mixture to a bowl and refrigerate for at least 2 hours.
4. Before serving top with whipped cream or coconut powder.

Servings: 2

Preparation Time: 5 minutes

Inactive Time: 2 hours

Nutrition Facts (per serving)

Calories 140,42

Total Fat 13,04g 20%

Total Carbohydrates 1,38g <1%

Fiber 0,01g <1%

Protein 4,34g 9%

Chocolate Mousse

Ingredients

1/4 cup of heavy cream

1 1/4 cup coconut cream

2 Tbsp of cocoa powder

3 Tbs of Erythritol (or Stevia)

1 Tbsp pure vanilla essence

shredded coconut, unsweetened

Directions

1. Scoop out the hardened coconut cream from the can, leaving the clear liquid behind, and place into a bowl. Add the heavy cream and combine with a hand mixer on low speed.
2. Add the remaining ingredients and mix on low speed for 2-3 minutes until the mix is thick.
3. Serve in individual ramekins sprinkled with unsweetened shredded coconut.

Servings: 4

Cooking Times: 15 minutes

Nutrition Facts (per serving)

Calories 305,19

Total Fat 31,91g 49%

Total Carbohydrates 6,97g 2%

Fiber 2,55g 10%

Protein 3,56g 7%

Strawberry Pudding

Ingredients

4 egg yolks

2 Tbsp butter

1/4 cup coconut flour

2 Tbsp heavy cream

1/4 cup strawberries

1/4 tsp baking powder

2 Tbsp coconut oil

2 tsp lemon juice

Zest 1 Lemon

2 Tbsp Erythritol

10 drops Liquid Stevia

Directions

1. Preheat oven to 350F.
2. In a bowl beat the egg yolks with electric mixer until they're pale in color. Add in Erythritol and 10 drops liquid Stevia. Beat again until fully combined.
3. Add in heavy cream, lemon juice, and the zest of 1 lemon. Add the coconut and butter. Beat well until no lumps are found.
4. Sift the dry ingredients over the wet ingredients, then mix well on a slow speed.
5. Distribute the strawberries evenly in the batter by pushing them into the top of the batter.
6. Bake for 20-25 minutes. Once finished, let cool for 5 minutes and serve.

Servings: 3

Cooking Times

Total Time: 35 minutes

Nutrition Facts (per serving)

Calories 258,65

Total Fat 23,46g 36%

Total Carbohydrates 9,3g 3%

Fiber 0,61g 2%

Protein 3,98g 8%

Kiwi Fiend Ice Cream

Ingredients

3 egg yolks

1 1/2 cup Kiwi, pureed

1 cup heavy cream

1/3 cup Erythritol

1/2 tsp pure vanilla extract

1/8 tsp chia seeds

Directions

1. In a sauce pan heat up the heavy cream. Add in 1/3 cup of erythritol to dissolve; simmer gently until erythritol is dissolved.
2. In a mixing bowl beat 3 egg yolks with an electric mixer. Add in a few tablespoons of your hot cream mixture at a time to the eggs while beating. Add in some pure vanilla extract and mix. Add in 1/8 tsp. of chia seeds.
3. Place your bowl into the freezer to chill for about 1-2 hours, stirring occasionally.
4. In a meanwhile puree the kiwi no more than 1-2 seconds. When the ice cream is chilled and getting a bit thicker, add in kiwi mixture to the chilled cream. Mix a bit.
5. Let the kiwi ice cream to chill at least 6-8 hours. Serve in chilled glasses.

Servings: 6

Cooking Times

Cooking Time: 15 minutes

Total Time: 8 hours and 15 minutes

Nutrition Facts (per serving)

Calories 192, 47

Total Fat 17,2g 26%

Total Carbohydrates 8,13g 3%

Fiber 1,46g 6%

Protein 2,69g 5%

Minty Avocado Lime Sorbet

Ingredients

1 cup coconut milk

2 avocados

1/4 mint leaves, chopped

1/4 cup powdered Erythritol

2 limes, juiced

1/4 tsp. liquid Stevia

Directions

1. Slice avocado half vertically through the flesh, making about 5 slices per half of an avocado. Use a spoon to carefully scoop out the pieces. Rest pieces on foil and squeeze juice of 1/2 lime over the tops.
2. Store avocado in freezer for at least 3 hours.
3. Using a spice grinder, powder Erythritol.
4. In a pan, bring coconut milk to a boil.
5. Zest the 2 limes you have while coconut milk is heating up. Add lime zest and continue to let the milk reduce in volume.
6. Remove and place the coconut milk into a container and store in the freezer.
7. Chop mint leaves. Remove avocados from freezer.
8. Add avocado, mint leaves, and juice from lime into the food processor. Pulse until a chunky consistency is achieved.
9. Pour coconut milk mixture over the avocados in the food processor. Add Liquid Stevia to this.
10. Pulse mixture together about 2-3 minutes.
11. Return to freezer to freeze, or serve immediately!

Servings: 6

Cooking Times

Total Time: 3 hours and 15 minutes

Nutrition Facts (per serving)

Calories 184, 18

Total Fat 17,26g 27%

Total Carbohydrates 9,65g 3%

Fiber 4,59g 18%

Protein 1,95g 4%

Morning Zephyr Cake

Ingredients

3 Tbsp. coconut oil

2 Tbsp. grounded flax seeds

8 Tbsp. almonds, grounded

1 cup Greek Yogurt

1 Tbsp. cocoa powder for dusting

1 cup heavy whipping cream

1 tsp. Baking Powder

1 tsp. Baking Soda

1 tsp. pure vanilla essence

1 pinch pink salt

1 cup Stevia or Erythritol sweetener

Directions

1. Pre-heat the oven at 350 F degrees.
2. In the blender first add the grounded almonds, grounded flax seeds and the baking powder and soda. Blend for a minute.
3. Add the salt, coconut oil and blend some more. Add the sweetener and blend for 2-3 minutes.
4. Add the Greek yogurt and blend for a minute or so, until a fine consistency is reached.
5. Take out the batter in a bowl and add the vanilla essence, and mix with a light hand.
6. Grease the baking dish and drop the batter in it.
7. Bake for 30 minutes. Let cool on a wire rack. Serve.

Servings: 8

Cooking Times

Total Time: 40 minutes

Nutrition Facts (per serving)

Calories 199, 84

Total Fat 20,69g 32%

Total Carbohydrates 3,22g 1%

Fiber 1,17g 5%

Protein 2,56g 5%

Peanut Butter Balls

Ingredients

2 eggs

2 1/2 cup of peanut butter

1/2 cup shredded coconut (unsweetened)

1/2 cup of Xylitol

1 Tbsp. of pure vanilla extract

Directions

1. Preheat oven to 320 F.
2. Mix all ingredients together by your hands.
3. After the ingredients are thoroughly mixed, roll into heaped tablespoon sized balls and press into a baking tray lined with baking paper.
4. Bake in the oven for 12 minutes or until the tops of the cookies are browning. When ready, let cool on a wire rack. Ready! Serve.

Servings: 16

Cooking Time: 22 minutes

Nutrition Facts (per serving)

Calories 254, 83

Total Fat 21,75g 33%

Total Carbohydrates 8,31g 3%

Fiber 2,64g 11%

Protein 10,98g 22%

Peppermint Chocolate Ice Cream

Ingredients

1/2 tsp. Peppermint extract

1 cup heavy cream

1 cup cheese cream

1 tsp. pure vanilla extract

1 tsp. Liquid Stevia extract

100% Dark Chocolate for topping

Directions

1. Place ice cream bowl in freezer per ice cream maker instructions. In a metal bowl, put all ingredients except chocolate and whisk well.
2. Put back in freezer for 5 minutes. Setup ice cream maker and add liquid.
3. Before serving, top the ice cream with chocolate shavings. Serve.

Servings: 3

Cooking Time: 35 minutes

Nutrition Facts (per serving)

Calories 286, 66

Total Fat 29,96g 46%

Total Carbohydrates 2,7g <1%

Fiber 0g 0%

Protein 2,6g 5%

Raspberry Chocolate Cream

Ingredients

1/2 cup 100% dark chocolate, chopped

1/4 cup of heavy cream

1/2 cup cream cheese, softened

2 Tbsp. sugar free Raspberry Syrup

1/4 cup Erythritol

Directions

1. In a double boiler melt chopped chocolate and the cream cheese. Add the Erythritol sweetener and continue to stir. Remove from heat, let cool and set aside.
2. When the cream has cooled add in heavy cream and Raspberry syrup and stir well.
3. Pour cream in a bowls or glasses and serve. Keep refrigerated.

Servings: 4

Cooking Time: 15 minutes

Nutrition Facts (per serving)

Calories 157, 67

Total Fat 13,51g 21%

Total Carbohydrates 7,47g 2%

Fiber 1g 4%

Protein 1,95g 4%

Raw Cacao Hazelnut Cookies

Ingredients

2 cups almond flour

1 cup chopped hazelnut

1/2 cup cacao powder

1/2 cup ground flax

3 Tbsp. coconut oil (melted)

1/3 cup water

1/3 cup Erythritol

1/4 tsp. liquid Stevia

Directions

1. In a bowl, mix almond flour and flax and cacao powder. Stir in oil, water, agave and vanilla. When it is well mixed, stir in chopped hazelnuts.
2. Form in to balls, press flat with palms and place on dehydrator screens.
3. Dehydrate 1 hour at 145, then reduce to 116 and dehydrate for at least 5 hours or until desired dryness is achieved.
4. Serve.

Servings: 24

Cooking Time: 6 hours

Nutrition Facts (per serving)

Calories 181, 12

Total Fat 15,69g 24%

Total Carbohydrates 8,75g 3%

Fiber 3,45g 14%

Protein 4,46g 9%

Sinless Pumpkin Cheesecake Muffins

Ingredients

1/2 cup pureed pumpkin

1 tsp. pumpkin pie spice

1/2 cup pecans, finely ground

1/2 cup cream cheese

1 Tbsp. coconut oil

1/2 tsp. pure vanilla extract

1/4 tsp. pure Yacon Syrup or Erythritol

Directions

1. Prepare a muffin tin with liners.
2. Place a small amount of ground pecans into every muffin tin and make a thin crust.
3. In a bowl, blend sweetener, spices, vanilla, coconut and the pumpkin puree. Add in the cream cheese and beat until the mixture is well combined.
4. Scoop about two tablespoons of filling mixture on top of each crust, and smooth around the edges.
5. Pop in the freezer for about 45 minutes.
6. Remove from the muffin tin and let sit for 10 minutes. Serve.

Servings: 6

Cooking Times

Total Time: 15 minutes

Nutrition Facts (per serving)

Calories 157, 34

Total Fat 15,52g 24%

Total Carbohydrates 3,94g 1%

Fiber 1,51g 6%

Protein 2,22g 4%

Hazelnut Biscuits with Arrowroot Tea

Ingredients

1 egg

1/2 cup hazelnuts

3 Tbsp. of coconut oil

2 cups almond flour

2 Tbsp. of arrowroot tea

2 tsp. ginger

1 Tbsp. cocoa powder

1/2 cup grapefruit juice

1 orange peel from a half orange

1/2 tsp. baking soda

1 pinch of salt

Directions

1. Preheat oven to 360 °F. Make arrowroot tea and let it cool.
2. In a food processor blend the hazelnuts. Add the remaining ingredients and continue blending until mixed well. With your hands form cookies with the batter.
3. Put the cookies on baking parchment paper, and bake for 30-35 minutes. When ready, remove tray from the oven and let cool.
4. Serve warm or cold.

Servings: 12

Cooking Times

Total Time: 50 minutes

Nutrition Facts (per serving)

Calories 224, 08

Total Fat 20,17g 31%

Total Carbohydrates 8,06g 3%

Fiber 3,25g 13%

Protein 6,36g 13%

Tartar Cookies

Ingredients

3 eggs

1/8 tsp. cream of tartar

1/3 cup cream cheese

1/8 tsp. salt

Some oil for greasing

Directions

1. Preheat oven to 300°F. Line the cookie sheet with parchment paper and grease with some oil.
2. Separate eggs from the egg yolks. Set both in different mixing bowls.
3. With an electric hand mixer, start beating the egg whites until super bubbly. Add in cream of tartar and beat until stiff peaks form.
4. In the egg yolk bowl, add in cream cheese and some salt. Beat until the egg yolks are pale yellow.
5. Merge the egg whites into the cream cheese mixture. Stir well.
6. Make cookies and place on the cookie sheet.
7. Bake for about 30-40 minutes. When ready, let them cool on a wire rack and serve.

Servings: 8

Cooking Times

Total Time: 35 minutes

Nutrition Facts (per serving)

Calories 59, 99

Total Fat 5,09g 8%

Total Carbohydrates 0,56g <1%

Fiber 0g 0%

Protein 2,93g 6%

Wild Strawberries Ice Cream

Ingredients

1/2 cup wild strawberries

1/3 cup cream cheese

1 cup heavy cream

1 Tbsp. lemon juice

1 tsp. pure vanilla extract

1/3 cup of your favorite sweetener

Ice cubes

Directions

1. Place all ingredients in a blender. Blend until all incorporate well.
2. Refrigerate for 2-3 hour before serving.

Servings: 4

Cooking Time: 5 minutes

Nutrition Facts (per serving)

Calories 176, 43

Total Fat 17,69g 27%

Total Carbohydrates 3,37g 1%

Fiber 0,39g 2%

Protein 1,9g 4%

Mini Lemon Cheesecakes

Ingredients

1 tablespoon lemon zest, grated

1 teaspoon lemon juice

½ teaspoon stevia powder or (Truvia)

1/4 cup coconut oil, softened

4 tablespoons unsalted butter, softened

4 ounces cream cheese (heavy cream)

Directions

1. Blend all ingredients together with a hand mixer or blender until smooth and creamy.

2. Prepare a cupcake or muffin tin with 6 paper liners.

3. Pour mixture into prepared tin and place in freezer for 2-3 hours or until firm.

4. Sprinkle cups with additional lemon zest. Or try using chopped nuts or shredded, unsweetened coconut.

Serves: 6

Cooking Time: 5 minutes

Nutrition Facts (per serving)

Calories: 196

Fat: 21.2 grams

Chocolate Layered Coconut Cups

Ingredients

<u>Bottom Layer:</u>

1/2 cup unsweetened, shredded coconut

3 tablespoons powdered sweetener such as Splenda or Truvia

1/2 cup coconut butter

1/2 cup coconut oil

<u>Top Layer:</u>

1 1/2 ounces cocoa butter

1 ounce unsweetened chocolate

1/4 cup cocoa powder

1/2 teaspoon vanilla extract

1/4 cup powdered sweetener such as Splenda or Truvia

Directions

1. Prepare a mini-muffin pan with 20 mini paper liners.
2. For the bottom layer:
3. Combine coconut butter and coconut oil in a small saucepan over low heat. Stir until smooth and melted then add the shredded coconut and powdered sweetener until combined.
4. Divide the mixture among prepared mini muffin cups and freeze until firm, about 30 minutes.
5. For the top layer:

6. Combine cocoa butter and unsweetened chocolate together in double boiler or a bowl set over a pan of simmering water. Stir until melted.

7. Stir in the powdered sweetener, then the cocoa powder and mix until smooth.

8. Remove from heat and stir in the vanilla extract.

9. Spoon chocolate topping over chilled coconut candies and let set, about 15 minutes.

10. Enjoy!

Serves: 10

Serving Size: 2 pieces

Nutrition Facts (per serving)
Calories: 240
Fat: 25 grams

Pumpkin Pie Chocolate Cups

Ingredients

For the crust:

3.5 ounces extra dark chocolate - 85% cocoa solids or more

2 tablespoons coconut oil

For the pie:

½ cup coconut butter

¼ cup coconut oil

2 teaspoons pumpkin pie spice mix

½ cup unsweetened pumpkin puree

2 tablespoons healthy low-carb sweetener

Optional: 15-20 drops liquid stevia for added sweetness

Directions

1. Place the chocolate and coconut oil in a double boiler or a glass bowl on top of a small saucepan filled with simmering water. Once completely melted, remove from the heat and set aside.

2. Prepare a mini muffin tin with 18 paper liners. Fill each of the 18 mini muffin cups with 2 teaspoons of the chocolate mixture. Place the chocolate in the fridge to set up for at least 10 minutes.

3. Place the coconut butter, coconut oil, sweetener and pumpkin spice mix into a bowl and melt just like you did the chocolate.

4. Add the pumpkin puree and mix until smooth and well combined.

5. Remove the muffin cups from the fridge and add a heaping teaspoon of the pumpkin & coconut mixture into every cup. Place back in the fridge and let it set for at least 30 minutes.

6. When done, keep refrigerated. Coconut oil and butter get very soft at room temperature. Store in the fridge for up to a week or freeze for up to 3 months. Enjoy!

Serves: 18

Serving Size: 1 mini pie

Nutrition Facts (per serving)

Calories: 110

Fat: 10.9 grams

Fudgy Slow Cooker Cake

Ingredients

1 1/2 cups almond flour

1/4 cup whey protein powder (chocolate, vanilla, and unflavored all work fine)

3/4 cup sugar substitute such as Swerve or Truvia

2/3 cup cocoa powder

2 teaspoons baking powder

1/4 teaspoon sea salt

1/2 cup butter, melted

4 large eggs

3/4 cup almond or coconut milk, unsweetened

1 teaspoon vanilla extract

1/2 cup chopped dark chocolate, 85% cocoa or higher

Whipped cream topping (optional):

1/2 cup heavy whipping cream

2 tablespoons sugar substitute

Directions

1. Grease the insert of a 6 quart slow cooker well with butter or coconut oil.

2. In a medium bowl, whisk together almond flour, sugar substitute, cocoa powder, whey protein powder, baking powder and salt.

3. Stir in butter, eggs, almond milk and vanilla extract until well combined, then fold in the chopped dark chocolate.

4. Pour into the greased slow cooker and cook on low for 2.5 to 3 hours. It will be gooey and like a pudding cake at 2.5 hours and little more cake like at 3 hours.

5. Turn slow cooker off and let cool for 20 to 30 minutes. Cut into pieces and serve warm.

6. Best when served with freshly whipped cream. To make this, mix the whipping cream and sugar substitute together with your stand mixer, or a hand mixer. Continue mixing until soft peaks form.

Serves: 10

Serving Size: 1/10th of cake

Nutrition Facts (per serving)
Calories: 275
Fat: 23

Easy Sticky Chocolate Fudge

Ingredients

1 cup coconut oil, softened

1/4 cup coconut milk (full fat, from a can)

1/4 cup cocoa powder

1 teaspoon vanilla extract

1/2 teaspoon sea salt

1-3 drops liquid stevia

Directions

1. With a hand mixer or stand mixer, whip the softened coconut oil and coconut milk together until smooth and glossy. About 6 minutes on high.

2. Add the cocoa powder, vanilla extract, sea salt, and one drop of liquid stevia to the bowl and mix on low until combined. Increase speed once everything is combined and mix for one minute. Taste fudge and adjust sweetness by adding additional liquid stevia, if desired.

3. Prepare a 9"x4" loaf pan by lining it with parchment paper.

4. Pour fudge into loaf pan and place in freezer for about 15, until just set.

5. Remove fudge and cut into 1" x 1" pieces. Store in an airtight container in the fridge or freezer.

Serves: 12

Nutrition Facts (per serving)

Calories: 172

Fat: 19.6 grams

Raspberry & Coconut Balls

Ingredients

1/2 cup coconut butter

1/2 cup coconut oil

1/2 cup freeze dried raspberries

1/2 cup unsweetened shredded coconut

1/4 powdered sugar substitute such as Swerve or Truvia

Directions

1. Line an 8"x8" pan with parchment paper.

2. In a food processor, coffee grinder, or blender, pulse the dried raspberries into a fine powder.

3. In a saucepan over medium heat, combine the coconut butter, coconut oil, coconut, and sweetener. Stir until melted and well combined.

4. Remove pan from heat and stir in raspberry powder.

5. Pour mixture into pan and refrigerate or freeze for several hours, or overnight.

6. Cut into 12 pieces and serve!

Serves: 12

Serving Size: 1 piece

Nutrition Facts (per serving)

Calories: 234

Fat: 23.6 grams

Strawberry Cheesecake Ice Cream Cups

Ingredients

1/2 strawberries, fresh or frozen, mashed well

3/4 cup cream cheese, softened

1/4 cup coconut oil, softened

10-15 drops liquid stevia

1 teaspoon vanilla extract

Directions

1. Combine all ingredients in a medium sized bowl and mix with a hand mixer until smooth and creamy. Can also be done in a food processor or high speed blender.)

2. Spoon the mixture into mini muffin silicon molds or small candy molds. Place in the freezer for about 2 hours or until set.

3. When done, unmold the fat bombs and place into a container. Keep in the freezer and enjoy any time!

Serves: 12

Serving Size: 1 bite

Nutrition Facts (per serving)

Calories: 67

Fat: 7.4 grams

Peppermint Patties

Ingredients

¾ cup melted coconut butter

¼ cup finely shredded, unsweetened coconut

2 tablespoons cacao powder

3 tablespoons coconut oil, melted

½ teaspoon pure peppermint extract

Directions

1. Mix together melted coconut butter, shredded coconut, 1 tablespoon of coconut oil and peppermint extract

2. Pour coconut butter mixture into mini muffin tins that have been lined with paper liners. Fill half way.

3. Place in refrigerator and allow to harden for about 15 minutes.

4. Mix together 2 tablespoons coconut oil and cacao powder.

5. Remove muffin tin from refrigerator and top each one with chocolate mixture.

6. Return to refrigerator until the chocolate has set.

7. When ready to eat, simply set the peppermint patty cups on the counter for about 5 minutes and unmold from muffin tin.

Serves: 12

Nutrition Facts (per serving)

Calories: 80

Fat: 7 grams

486

Buttery Pecan Delights

Ingredients

8 pecan halves

1 tablespoon unsalted butter, softened

2 ounces neufchâtel cheese

1 teaspoon orange zest, finely grated

pinch of sea salt

Directions

1. Toast the pecans at 350 degrees Fahrenheit for 5-10 minutes, check often to prevent burning.

2. Mix the butter, neufchâtel cheese, and orange zest until smooth and creamy.

3. Spread the butter mixture between the cooled pecan halves and sandwich together.

4. Sprinkle with sea salt and enjoy!

Serves: 2

Serving Size: 2 pecan sandwiches

Nutrition Facts (per serving)

Calories: 163

Fat: 16 grams

Fudge Oh So Chocolate

Ingedients

1 cup coconut oil, softened

1/4 cup coconut milk (full fat, from a can)

1/2 teaspoon sea salt

1-3 drops liquid stevia

1/4 cup cocoa powder

1 teaspoon vanilla extract

Directions

1. With a hand mixer or stand mixer, whip the softened coconut oil and coconut milk together until smooth and glossy. About 6 minutes on high.

2. Add the cocoa powder, vanilla extract, sea salt, and one drop of liquid stevia to the bowl and mix on low until combined. Increase speed once everything is combined and mix for one minute. Taste fudge and adjust sweetness by adding additional liquid stevia, if desired.

3. Prepare a 9"x4" loaf pan by lining it with parchment paper.

4. Pour fudge into loaf pan and place in freezer for about 15, until just set.

5. Remove fudge and cut into 1" x 1" pieces. Store in an airtight container in the fridge or freezer.

Serves: 12

Nutrition Facts (per serving)

Calories: 172

Fat: 19.6 grams

Cinna-Bun Balls

Ingredients

1 cup coconut butter

1 teaspoon vanilla extract

1 cup full fat coconut milk (from a can)

1 cup unsweetened coconut shreds

1/2 teaspoon cinnamon

1/2 teaspoon nutmeg

1 teaspoon sugar substitute such as Splenda

Directions

1. Combine all ingredients except the shredded coconut together in double boiler or a bowl set over a pan of simmering water. Stir until everything is melted and combined.

2. Remove bowl from heat and place in the fridge until the mixture has firmed up and can be rolled into balls.

3. Form the mixture into 1″ balls, a small cookie scoop is helpful for doing this.

4. Roll each ball in the shredded coconut until well coated.

5. Serve and enjoy! Store in the fridge.

Serves: 10

Nutrition Facts (per serving)

Calories: 273

Fat: 30.9 grams

Vanilla Mousse Cups

Ingredients

8 ounces (1 block) cream cheese, softened

1/2 cup sugar substitute such as Swerve or Truvia (Stevia)

1 1/2 teaspoons vanilla extract

dash of sea salt

1/2 cup heavy whipping cream

Directions

1. Add the first four ingredients to a food processor or blender.

2. Blend until combined.

3. With blender running, slowly add the heavy cream.

4. Continue to blend until thickened, about 1-2 minutes. Consistency should be mousse like.

5. Prepare a cupcake or muffin tin with 6 paper liners and portion the mixture into the cups.

6. Chill in the fridge until set and enjoy!

Serves: 6

Nutrition Facts (per serving)

Calories: 199

Fat: 20.2 grams

Rich & Creamy Ice Cream

Ingredients

4 whole pastured eggs

4 yolks from pastured eggs

⅓ cup melted cocoa butter

⅓ cup melted coconut oil

15-20 drops liquid stevia

⅓ cup cocoa powder

¼ cup MCT oil

2 teaspoons pure vanilla extract

8-10 ice cubes

Directions

1. Add all ingredients but the ice cubes into the jug of your high speed blender. Blend on high for 2 minutes, until creamy.

2. While the blender is running, remove the top portion of the lid and drop in 1 ice cube at a time, allowing the blender to run about 10 seconds between each ice cube.

3. Once all of the ice has been added, pour the cold mixture into a 9×5″ loaf pan and place in the freezer. Set the timer for 30 minutes before taking out to stir. Repeat this process for 2-3 hours, until desired consistency is met.

4. Serve immediately. Top with chopped nuts or shaved dark chocolate, if desired.

5. Store covered in the freezer for up to a week.

Serves: 5

Serving Size: 1 cup

Nutrition Facts (per serving)

Calories: 431

Fat: 44.3

English Toffee Treats

Ingredients

1 cup coconut oil

2 tablespoons butter

1/2 block cream cheese, softened

3/4 tablespoons cocoa powder

1/2 cup creamy, natural peanut butter

3 tablespoons Davinci Gourmet Sugar Free English Toffee Syrup

Directions

1. Combine all ingredients in a saucepan over medium heat.

2. Stir until everything is smooth, melted, and combined.

3. Pour mixture into small candy molds or mini muffin tins lined with paper liners.

4. Freeze or refrigerate until set and enjoy!

5. Store in an airtight container in the fridge.

Serves: 24

Serving Size: 1 piece

Nutrition Facts (per serving)

Calories: 142

Fat: 15 grams

Fudgy Peanut Butter Squares

Ingredients

1 cup all natural creamy peanut butter

1 cup coconut oil

1/4 cup unsweetened vanilla almond milk

a pinch of coarse sea salt

1 teaspoon vanilla extract

2 teaspoons liquid stevia (optional)

Directions

1. In a microwave safe bowl, soften the peanut butter and coconut oil together. (About 1 minute on med-low heat.)

2. Combine the softened peanut butter and coconut oil with the remaining ingredients into a blender or food processor.

3. Blend until thoroughly combined.

4. Pour into a 9X4" loaf pan that has been lined with parchment paper.

5. Refrigerate until set. About 2 hours.

6. Enjoy!

Serves: 12

Nutrition Facts (per serving)

Calories: 287

Fat: 29.7

Almond Butter Balls

Ingredients

2 1/2 cup almond butter

1/2 cup shredded coconut (unsweetened)

2 eggs

1/2 cup Stevia sweetener

1 Tbsp. pure vanilla extract

Directions

1. Preheat oven to 320 F. Line square baking tray with baking paper.
2. Place all ingredients in a bowl. Knead the mixture by your hands.
3. After the ingredients are mixed, roll into heaped teaspoon sized balls and place into a baking tray.
4. Bake in the oven for 12 minutes or until the tops of the cookies are browning. Let cool on a wire rack. Serve.

Servings: 24

Cooking Time: 22 minutes

Nutrition Facts (per serving)

Total Carbs: 5,6g

Protein: 7,3g

Total Fat: 14,5g

Calories: 171

Cheesy Hazelnut Morsels

Ingredients

1/2 cup ground hazelnuts

1/4 cup hazelnut butter

1 cup cream cheese

1/4 cup cocoa powder

2 Tbsp.p Sugar free Hazelnut syrup

Natural sweetener of your cheese, to taste

Directions

1. In a large bowl, place the softened cream cheese (on room temperature) and hazelnut butter. Add in all other ingredients (except the ground hazelnuts).
2. With a wooden spoon to blend the cream cheese, cocoa powder, butter, syrup and sweetener.
3. In a bowl place the ground hazelnuts. Roll the cream cheese mixture into 16 balls. Dip each ball into the ground hazelnuts.
4. Refrigerate for at least 2-3 hours.

Servings: 16

Cooking Time: 15 minutes

Nutrition Facts (per serving)

Total Carbohydrates: 3,4g

Dietary Fiber: 1,4g

Net Carbs: 1,2g

Protein: 3,2g

Total Fat: 11,6g

Calories: 122

Choco Mint Hazelnut Sticks

Ingredients

4 Tbsp. cocoa powder

1 cup shredded coconut

1 cup hazelnuts

1 tsp. peppermint extract

6 Tbsp. coconut oil, melted

4 Tbsp. almond butter

3/4 cup Stevia sweetener (or some other natural sweetener of your choice)

1 tsp. vanilla extract

pinch of salt

Directions

1. In a large bowl stir together the coconut oil, cacao powder, almond butter, sweetener, vanilla, peppermint extract and salt. Chop the hazelnuts in a food processor.
2. Heat the mixture slowly on low heat over simmering water (double boiler) for 5 to 10 minutes until all ingredients are combined well.
3. Add hazelnuts and shredded coconut to the melted chocolate mixture and stir together.
4. Pour in a dish lined with parchment and freeze until chocolate is set then cut into sticks.

Servings: 12

Cooking Times

Total Time: 20 minutes

Nutrition Facts (per serving)

Total Carbohydrates: 5,6g

Dietary Fiber: 2,4g

Net Carbs: 2g

Protein: 3g

Total Fat: 17g

Calories: 174

Chocolate Bomb Cookies

Ingredients

1 Tbsp. cacao powder

2 Tbsp chocolate protein powder

4 Tbsp. coconut milk

2 Tbsp. coconut flour

2 Tbsp. coconut, shredded

1 Tbsp. cacao nibs

Topping

1 tsp. coconut oil, softened

2/3 cup coconut butter, softened

Directions

1. In a bowl combine all ingredients (except ingredients for coating). Whisk 2-3 minutes until well combined.
2. Spoon out mixture into small molds.
3. Place molds in refrigerator for 30 minutes.
4. In a meanwhile prepare coating. In a bowl, mix coconut oil with coconut butter. Remove molds from refrigerator and cover with coating
5. Place back to refrigerator until coating has hardened, about 1 hour.

Servings: 10

Cooking Times

Total Time: 10 minutes

Nutrition Facts (per serving)

Total Carbohydrates: 2,55g

Dietary Fiber: 1g

Net Carbs: 0,71g

Protein: 1g

Total Fat: 14,47g

Calories: 138

Chocolate Peanut Butter Balls

Ingredients

1/2 stick butter, softened

1/2 cup natural peanut butter

2 Tbsp. coconut flour

2 Tbsp. vanilla whey protein powder

1/2 cup broken up sugar free chocolate bars, melted

1 tsp. organic vanilla extract

1 1/2 cup powdered Xylitol (or some other natural sweetener)

Directions

1. In a bowl, mix peanut butter and butter. Beat the butter with an electric hand mixer, beat together butter until smooth.
2. Add in vanilla extract and protein powder to peanut butter mixture, and then mix well.
3. Add in powdered Xylitol sweetener and mix well.
4. On a working surface, roll the dough into 24 two-bite sized balls. Place balls on a pan lined with a parchment paper.
5. Sprinkle each ball with chocolate. Refrigerate for at least 2 hours.

Servings: 12

Cooking Times

Total Time: 10 minutes

Nutrition Facts (per serving)

Total Carbohydrates: 5,16g

Dietary Fiber: 1,02g

Net Carbs: 2,54g

Protein: 3g

Total Fat: 12g

Calories: 126

Choco-Orange Walnut Muffin Bombs

Ingredients

1 1/2 cup walnuts, chopped

4.40 oz. dark chocolate, 100% cocoa

1 tsp. natural orange extract

1 tsp. fresh orange peel

4 Tbsp.p extra virgin coconut oil

15-20 drops of liquid Stevia

1 tsp. cinnamon

Directions

1. In a heated container of water (water bath) melt the chocolate stirring slightly. Add liquid Stevia, coconut oil and cinnamon. Mix well.
2. Add fresh orange peel and natural orange extract. Add chopped walnuts and mix in well.
3. When ready, with teaspoon place the mixture into small paper muffin.
4. Place in the fridge until solid, at least 4-6 hours.

Servings: 18

Cooking Times

Total Time: 20 minutes

Nutrition Facts (per serving)

Total Carbohydrates: 5g

Dietary Fiber: 1,5g

Net Carbs: 3g

Protein: 13g

Total Fat: 13g

Calories: 131

Cinnamon Storms

Ingredients

1 cup coconut milk

1 cup almond butter

1 tsp. pure vanilla extract

3/4 tsp. cinnamon

1/2 tsp. nutmeg

1 tsp. natural sweetener to your taste)

1 cup coconut shreds

Directions

1. In a double boiler over medium heat place all the ingredients (except shredded coconut). Stir all the time to melt and combine well.
2. When ready, remove from the heat. Let cool for 5-6 minutes. Place the bowl in the fridge about 45 minutes until hard.
3. In a bowl put the coconut shreds. Roll the coconut-cinnamon mixture into one inch balls and roll them through the coconut shreds.
4. Place the balls on a serving plate and refrigerate for 2-3 hours.

Servings: 12

Cooking Times

Preparation Time: 1 hour and 30 minutes

Nutrition Facts (per serving)

Total Carbohydrates: 1,6g

Dietary Fiber: 0,5g

Net Carbs: 0,2g

Protein: 1g

Total Fat: 20g

Calories: 184

Creamy Orange Bites

Ingredients

1/2 cup heavy whipping cream

1/2 cup cream cheese

1/2 cup coconut oil, melted

1 tsp. pure orange extract

10 drops Liquid Stevia (or the natural sweetener of your choice)

Directions

1. In an immersion blender place all ingredients. Blend until corporate well.
2. Add in orange extract and liquid Stevia and mix together with a spoon.
3. Spread the batter mixture into a silicone tray, or in paper muffins trays.
4. Refrigerate for 2 hours. Before serving remove from silicone tray and serve. Keep refrigerated.

Servings: 14

Cooking Time: 10 minutes

Nutrition Facts (per serving)

Total Carbohydrates: 0,5g

Protein: 1g

Total Fat: 14g

Calories: 127

Coco-Nut Bites

Ingredients

1 1/2 cup flaked coconut, unsweetened

1 cup coconut oil

1 cup extra virgin coconut oil

1 tsp. cinnamon powder

1/8 tsp. salt

2 Tbsp. of powdered Erythritol

Directions

1. Preheat the oven 350 F.
2. Arrange evenly the flaked coconut on a rectangular baking tray. Place in the oven and toast for 8 minutes strictly. Let cool 2-3 minutes.
3. Transfer baked coconut into a blender and pulse until get a smooth and runny consistency.
4. Add the softened coconut oil, vanilla, Erythritol, salt and cinnamon. Blend well.
5. Pour the mixture with the tablespoon into ice cube tray to get 12 servings. Refrigerate for at least 2-3 hours.
6. Ready. Serve and enjoy! Keep refrigerated.

Servings: 12

Cooking Times

Total Time: 15 minutes

Nutrition Facts (per serving)

Total Carbohydrates: 1,5g

Dietary Fiber: 1g

Net Carbs: 0,6g

Protein: 0,4g

Total Fat: 13g

Calories: 114

Easy Choco Blueberry Squares

Ingredients

5 Tbsp. butter

3 Tbsp. coconut oil

2 Tbsp. sugar-free Blueberry syrup

2 Tbsp. cocoa powder

Directions

1. In a sauce pan add all ingredients and cook over low heat until chocolate sauce texture.
2. Pour into mold and freeze for at least 3 hours.
3. Before serving unmold and enjoy.

Servings: 6

Cooking Time: 15 minutes

Nutrition Facts (per serving)

Total Carbohydrates: 1g

Dietary Fiber: 0,6g

Net Carbs: 0, 05

Protein: 0,5g

Total Fat: 17g

Calories: 148

Easy Jello Balls

Ingredients

1 cup cream cheese

1/4 cup coconut butter

1 package of sugar free jello

Directions

1. In a small bowl put the jello powder.
2. In a separate bowl, mix together cream cheese and coconut butter.
3. Take a teaspoon of batter, roll into a ball in your hands and then roll in the jello powder. Make 16 balls.
4. Cover with plastic wrap and place in the fridge.

Servings: 8

Cooking Time 10 minutes

Nutrition Facts (per serving)

Total Carbohydrates: 1,20g

Net Carbs: 1g

Protein: 2g

Total Fat: 16g

Calories: 150g

Gingery Coconut Fat Bomb

Ingredients

1 tsp. dried (powdered) ginger

0.8 oz. shredded coconut (unsweetened)

1/3 cup coconut oil, softened

1/3 cup coconut butter, softened

1 tsp. granulated sweetener of choice, to taste

Directions

1. In a deep bowl, mix shredded coconut, coconut oil, coconut butter, sweetener and dried powdered ginger.
2. Pour the ginger mixture into ice block trays and refrigerate for 1 hour to solidify.

Servings: 10

Cooking Time: 5 minutes

Nutrition Facts (per serving)

Total Carbohydrates: 2,5g

Net Carbs: 0,3g

Protein:

Total Fat: 14,5g

Calories: 134

Homemade Almond Butter

Ingredients

3 cups almonds (no salt added)

1 tsp. Himalayan salt

1 tsp. cinnamon

1 vanilla pod or bean, halved and seeds removed

2 Tbsp. Stevia powder or Erythritol sweetener

Directions

1. Preheat oven to 360F degrees. Place almonds in a baking pan and bake for 10-12 minutes. Stir occasionally to not burn.
2. Transfer the almonds in a food processor and add remaining ingredients.
3. Process for 15 minutes above. This process takes a time so, you have to be patient. Pour the almond butter to a glass container and store in the refrigerator.

Servings: 14

Cooking Times

Total Time: 40 minutes

Nutrition Facts (per serving)

Total Carbohydrates: 5,5g

Dietary Fiber: 2,8g

Net Carbs: 1.3g

Protein: 5g

Total Fat: 13,5g

Calories: 153g

Almond Cookies

Ingredients

1 cup almonds, chopped

1 cup butter, softened

2 1/4 cups almond flour

1 1/4 cup cocoa powder

3 1/2 Tbsp. coconut flour

2 eggs

3/4 cup Stevia powder

2 tsp. vanilla extract

1/2 tsp. baking soda

1/4 tsp. sea salt

Directions

1. Preheat oven to 340F degrees.
2. In a bowl, whisk butter and sweetener. Add the eggs, coconut oil and vanilla extract.
3. In a separate bowl, mix together the baking soda, almond flour, coconut flour, cocoa powder and salt.
4. Combine the eggs mixture to the flour mixture. Pour dough in a greased baking pan. Sprinkle dough with chopped almond over top.
5. Bake for 15-18 minutes. Let cool and cut into chunks. Serve.

Servings: 16

Cooking Times

Total Time: 25 minutes

Nutrition Facts (per serving)

Total Carbohydrates: 3,35g

Dietary Fiber: 1g

Net Carbs: 0,5g

Protein: 2,9g

Total Fat: 17g

Calories: 171

Chocolate & Hazelnut Squares

Ingredients

1/2 cup hazelnuts, chopped

1 cup whipped cream

1/4 cup cocoa butter

2 Tbsp. cocoa powder, unsweetened

2 Tbsp. Stevia sweetener

Crushed walnuts (optional extra)

Directions

1. In a bowl, melt cocoa butter at room temperature.
2. When ready, add in cocoa powder, Stevia powder and mix well until all ingredients are well blended. Add in chopped hazelnuts and stir well.
3. Finally, add whipping cream and mix well.
4. Pour the hazelnut mixture in squared molds and let cool. (ice trays work just fine)
5. Refrigerate for 1 - 2 hours. Dress with crushed walnuts if so desired Serve.

Servings: 6

Cooking Times

Total Time: 15 minutes

Nutrition Facts (per serving)

Total Carbohydrates: 3,8g

Dietary Fiber: 1,3g

Net Carbs: 0,5g

Protein: 2g

Total Fat: 16,5g

Calories: 160

Low Carb Lime Balls

Ingredients

fresh lime zest from 2 organic limes

1 cup extra virgin coconut oil, softened

3/4 cup coconut butter, softened

20 drops Erythritol extract (or some other natural sweetener of your choice)

pinch of salt

Directions

1. Soft the coconut butter and coconut oil on room temperature.
2. Zest the organic limes.
3. In a bowl mix all the ingredients in a bowl and stir well. Make sure that lime zest and Erythritol extract are distributed evenly.
4. Prepare 16 mini muffin cups.
5. Refrigerate for 2 hours. Ready. Keep refrigerated.

Servings: 16

Cooking Times

Total Time: 10 minutes

Nutrition Facts (per serving)

Total Carbohydrates: 0,9g

Dietary Fiber: 0,3g

Net Carbs: 0,15g

Protein: 0,2g

Total Fat: 12,5g

Calories: 109

Lemon Coconut Balls

Ingredients

1/4 cup shredded coconut, unsweetened,

1 cup cream cheese

1 Tbsp. pure lemon extract

Natural sweetener of your choice, to taste

1/4 cup butter

Directions

1. In a bowl, combine cream cheese, natural sweetener and lemon extract. Blend all ingredients together well with mixing spoon. Place bowl in refrigerator for 15-20 minutes.
2. In a bowl place unsweetened shredded coconut. Roll lemon batter into 16 equal balls.
3. Dip each ball into coconut and place on a serving pan. Refrigerate for 3-4 hours at least. Serve.

Servings: 12

Cooking Time: 15 minutes

Nutrition Facts (per serving)

Total Carbohydrates: 1g

Protein: 1,3g

Total Fat: 12g

Calories: 106

Heavenly Lemon Quads with Coconut Cream

Ingredients

Base

3/4 cup coconut flakes

2 Tbsp. coconut oil

1 Tbsp. ground almonds

Cream

5 eggs

1/2 lemon juice

1 Tbsp. coconut flour

1/2 cup Stevia sweetener

Directions

For the Base

1. Preheat oven to 360F.
2. In a bowl put all base ingredients and with clean hands mix everything well until soft.
3. With coconut oil grease a rectangle oven dish. Pour dough in a baking pan. Bake for 15 minutes until golden brown. Set aside to cool.

For the Cream

1. In a bowl or blender, whisk together: eggs, lemon juice, coconut flour and sweetener. Pour over the baked caked evenly.
2. Put pan in the oven and bake 20 minutes more.
3. When ready refrigerate for at least 6 hours. Cut in cubes and serve.

Servings: 8

Cooking Times

Total Time: 1 hour and 5 minutes

Nutrition Facts (per serving)

Total Carbohydrates: 4g

Dietary Fiber: 2,25g

Net Carbs: 1,4g

Protein: 5g

Total Fat: 15g

Calories: 129

Macadamia Cacao Cookies

Ingredients

1 cup macadamia nuts, chopped

1/2 cup cacao powder

2 cups almond flour

1/2 cup ground flax

3 Tbsp. coconut oil (melted)

1/3 cup Stevia or natural sweetener of your choice

1/3 cup water

1/2 tsp. pure vanilla extract

Directions

1. In a bowl, mix almond flour and flax and cacao powder. Stir in oil, water, sweetener and vanilla. When it is well mixed, stir in chopped hazelnuts.
2. Form the mixture into balls, press flat with palms and place on dehydrator screens.
3. Dehydrate 1 hour at 145, then reduce to 116 and dehydrate for at least 5 hours or until desired dryness is achieved.

Servings: 24

Cooking Times

Total Time: 6 hours

Nutrition Facts (per serving)

Total Carbohydrates: 7g

Dietary Fiber: 3g

Net Carbs: 3, 4

Protein: 3,5g

Total Fat: 13g

Calories: 143

Minty Galettes

Ingredients

3 cup coconut butter, melted

1 cup coconut, shredded

3 Tbsp.p coconut oil melted

3/4 tsp. pure peppermint extract

2 Tbsp.p cacao powder

Directions

1. In a bowl, mix together, 1 tablespoon of coconut oil and peppermint extract, shredded coconut and melted coconut butter.
2. Pour coconut butter mixture into mini muffin tins by filling half way. Put in refrigerator for about 20 minutes.
3. In a separate bowl mix together 2 tablespoons coconut oil and cacao powder.
4. After 20 minutes remove muffin tin from refrigerator and pour each with cacao mixture.
5. Return to refrigerator for 3-4 hours. Ready!

Servings: 18

Cooking Times

Total Time: 20 minutes

Nutrition Facts (per serving)

Total Carbohydrates: 0,5g

Dietary Fiber: 0,3g

Net Carbs: 0,1g

Protein: 0,25g

Total Fat: 11g

Calories: 93

Peppermint Ice Cream Balls

Ingredients

1 1/4 cup seed butter

1 tsp. peppermint extract

1 1/2 cups coconut oil

1/2 cup sweetener (liquid or granulated)

2 tsp. organic vanilla extract

1/4 tsp. salt

Directions

1. First, in a small saucepan melt the coconut oil.
2. In a blender add all remaining ingredients and add melted coconut oil. Blend it until smooth well.
3. With the teaspoon grab the coconut mixture and make the 25 coconut balls.
4. Place the balls into a baking sheet and freeze until solid. Keep refrigerated.

Servings: 25

Cooking Times

Total Time: 10 minutes

Nutrition Facts (per serving)

Total Carbohydrates: 8g

Dietary Fiber: 1.2g

Net Carbs: 0,25g

Protein: 2.25g

Total Fat: 19g

Calories: 202

Pistachio Masala Delights

Ingredients

1 cup almond butter, melted

1/4 cup ghee

1 cup coconut oil

1/2 cup cocoa butter

1/4 cup pistachio nuts

1 Tbsp. coconut milk

1 Tbsp.p pure vanilla extract

2 tsp. Masala chai (a flavored tea beverage made by brewing black tea with a mixture of aromatic Indian spices and herbs)

Directions

1. In a small saucepan melt the cocoa butter over LOW heat.
2. In a large bowl add all ingredients (except the cocoa butter and pistachios).
3. Use a hand mixer and mix well (on HIGH) all ingredients until the mixture combine evenly. Add in the melted butter and continue to blend for 1-2 minutes more.
4. Transfer the mixture to greased and paper lined pan. Sprinkle with chopped pistachios and refrigerate for at least 5 hours.

Servings: 32

Cooking Times

Total Time: 15 minutes

Nutrition Facts (per serving)

Total Carbohydrates: 0,4g

Dietary Fiber: 0,1g

Net Carbs: 0,1g

Protein: 0, 27

Total Fat: 17g

Calories: 147

Raspberry Heaven Squares

Ingredients

3 Tbsp. heavy cream

1/4 cup coconut oil, melted

8 oz. cream cheese, softened

1/4 cup coconut oil, melted

3 tsp. raspberry extract

1/2 cup powdered Erythritol

pinch salt

few drops of natural red food coloring

Directions

1. Prepare the parchment lined baking sheet.
2. In a bowl, with the hand mixer, blend the cream cheese and sweetener together.
3. Add the raspberry extract, natural food coloring cream, salt and raspberry extract and continue to blend.
4. Add in the coconut oil and continue to blend until it's smooth and creamy.
5. Refrigerate this mixture for 1 hour.
6. When ready, make 48 small balls from batter and place into a prepared parchment lined baking sheet. Place it in a freezer for 2 hours.

Servings: 18

Cooking Times

Total Time: 15 minutes

Nutrition Facts (per serving)

Total Carbohydrates: 0,6g

Dietary Fiber: 0g

Net Carbs: 0.4g

Protein: 0, 77

Total Fat: 12g

Calories: 101

Slow Cooker Pecan Nuts

Ingredients

2 cups Pecans nuts, halves

4 Tbsp. almond butter

1 cup Stevia or any other natural sweetener

1/4 tsp. ground ginger

1/4 tsp. ground allspice

1 1/2 tsp. ground cinnamon

Directions

1. In a 4-quart Slow Cooker stir the Pecans nuts halves and almond butter until combined.
2. Add Stevia or any natural sweetener of your choice and stir well.
3. Transfer to a bowl, combine spices and sprinkle over nuts.
4. Cover and cook on HIGH for 15 minutes. Turn to LOW and cook uncovered for about 2 hours, or until the nuts are a little crispy.

Servings: 8

Cooking Times

Total Time: 2 hours and 15 minutes

Nutrition Facts (per serving)

Total Carbohydrates: 3,6g

Dietary Fiber: 2,3g

Net Carbs: 0,88g

Protein: 2,9g

Total Fat: 14g

Calories: 140

Strawberry Cream-cakes

Ingredients

5 strawberries

1/2 cup heavy cream

5 Tbsp. butter

5 Tbsp. coconut oil

3 Tbsp. Truvia (or any favorite sweetener)

1 peace dark 100%, sugar free chocolate

Directions

1. In a bowl, mix heavy cream and the strawberries.
2. With a help of an immersion blender, blend together heavy cream and strawberries.
3. In a separate bowl, add granulated sweetener and the butter; melt butter mixture in the microwave about 30 seconds.
4. Add the butter mixture to a heavy cream and strawberries and blend well.
5. Spoon mixture into your favorite molds. Freeze at least 30 minutes; the longer, the better.
6. Remove mixture from the mold, place on wax paper and melt one piece sugar free chocolate.
7. Pour melted chocolate over the cream and return to freezer for another 30 minutes.

Servings: 12

Cooking Times

Total Time: 1 hour and 10 minutes

Nutrition Facts (per serving)

Total Carbohydrates: 0,6g

Dietary Fiber: 0,08g

Net Carbs: 0,2g

Protein: 0,3gr

Total Fat: 16g

Calories: 138

Strawberry Muffins

Ingredients

3/4 cup cream cheese, softened

1/4 cup butter, softened

1/2 cup strawberries, fresh or frozen

1 Tbsp.p pure vanilla extract

10–15 drops liquid Stevia

Directions

1. In a mixing bowl, place the butter and the cream cheese and eave at room temperature (about 45min) until softened. Do not microwave the butter!
2. In a separate bowl place the strawberries and mash using a fork.
3. Add the liquid Stevia and vanilla extract and mix well. Add the strawberries to the bowl with softened butter and cream cheese. Whisk until all ingredients are well combined.
4. Pour the strawberry mixture into muffin silicon molds. Place in the freezer for about 3-4 hours.
5. Before serving, unmold the strawberry muffins and place on a serving dish. Keep refrigerated.

Servings: 10

Cooking Times

Total Time: 10 minutes

Nutrition Facts (per serving)

Total Carbohydrates: 1,5g

Dietary Fiber: 0,2g

Net Carbs: 1,1g

Protein: 1,15g

Total Fat: 11g

Calories: 107

Walnuts Choco Fat Bombs

Ingredients

1/3 cup heavy cream

1/2 cup cocoa butter

1/2 cup pecans, roughly chopped

1/2 cup coconut oil

4 Tbsp. cocoa powder, unsweetened

4 Tbsp. Swerve, Stevia or Erythritol sweetener

Directions

1. In a microwave dish, place cocoa butter and coconut oil together. Use the defrost setting on your microwave and melt in microwave stove for 10-15 seconds.
2. Add in cocoa powder and whisk well. Pour mixture into a blender with sweetener and cream and blend for 3-4 minutes.
3. Place silicone molds onto a sheet pan and fill halfway with walnuts.
4. Pour the mixture with walnuts and place in refrigerator for 6 hours.

Servings: 10

Cooking Times

Total Time: 10 minutes

Nutrition Facts (per serving)

Total Carbohydrates: 2,23g

Dietary Fiber: 1,25g

Net Carbs: 0,25g

Protein: 1g

Total Fat: 29g

Calories: 150

Almond Butter Cake with Choco Sauce

Ingredients

1 cup almond butter or soaked almonds

1/4 cup almond milk, unsweetened

1 cup coconut oil

2 tsp liquid Stevia sweetener to taste

Topping: Chocolate Sauce

4 Tbsp cocoa powder, unsweetened

2 Tbsp almond butter

2 Tbsp Stevia sweetener

Directions

1. Melt the coconut oil in room temperature.
2. Add all ingredients in a bowl and blend well until combined.
3. Pour the almond butter mixture into a parchment lined platter.
4. Place in refrigerator for 3 hours.
5. In a bowl, whisk all topping ingredients together. Pour over the almond cake after it's been set. Cut into cubes and serve.

Servings: 12

Cooking Times

Total Time: 5 minutes

Nutrition Facts (per serving)

Total Carbohydrates: 9,8g

Dietary Fiber: 2g

Net Carbs:2,4g

Protein: 5,8g

Total Fat: 23,3g

Calories: 273

Choco Almond Candy's

Ingredients

3 Tbsp cocoa powder, unsweetened

1 cup almond butter

1 cup organic coconut oil

3-4 Tbsp sweetener to taste

Splash of almond extract (optional)

Directions

1. In a saucepan over medium heat, melt coconut oil and almond butter. Stir in cocoa powder and sweetener of zour choice. Remove from heat and add almond extract.
2. Pour almond mixture into silicone candy molds. Freeze or refridgerate until set.
3. Before using remove from molds and store in a fridge in an air tight container.

Servings: 24

Cooking Time: 10 minutes

Nutrition Facts (per serving)

Total Carbohydrates: 0,4g

Dietary Fiber: 1,22g

Net Carbs: 0g

Protein: 0,5g

Total Fat: 9,6g

Calories: 75

Chocolate-Coconut Layered Cups

Ingredients

Bottom Layer:

1/2 cup coconut butter

1/2 cup coconut oil

1/2 cup unsweetened, shredded coconut

3 Tbsp powdered sweetener such as Splenda or Truvia

Top Layer:

1/2 cup cocoa butter

1 oz unsweetened chocolate

1/4 cup powdered sweetener such as Splenda or Truvia

1/4 cup cocoa powder

1/2 tsp vanilla extract

Directions

1. Prepare a mini-muffin pan with 20 mini paper liners.
2. **For the bottom layer:**
3. Combine coconut butter and coconut oil in a small saucepan over low heat. Stir until smooth and melted then add the shredded coconut and powdered sweetener until combined.
4. Divide the mixture among prepared mini muffin cups and freeze until firm, about 30 minutes.
5. **For the top layer:**
6. Combine cocoa butter and unsweetened chocolate together in double boiler or a bowl set over a pan of simmering water. Stir until melted.

7. Stir in the powdered sweetener, then the cocoa powder and mix until smooth.
8. Remove from heat and stir in the vanilla extract.
9. Spoon chocolate topping over chilled coconut candies and let set, about 15 minutes.
10. Enjoy!

Servings: 10

Nutrition Facts (per serving)

Total Carbohydrates: 2,7g

Dietary Fiber: 1,5g

Net Carbs: 0,35g

Protein: 1g

Total Fat: 27,5g

Calories: 247

Author Notes

Chocolate contains antioxidants known as polyphenols. Polyphenols play an important role in the prevention of degenerative diseases such as cancer and cardiovascular diseases.

Chocolate-Walnut Squares

Ingredients

1/2 cup coconut oil

1 oz cocoa powder

1 Tbs sugar substitute

1 oz walnut pieces

1 Tbs tahini paste

Walnut halves for topping the fat bombs

Directions

1. Warm the coconut oil in the microwave until melted.
2. Add the remaining ingredients and stir until well combined.
3. Pour into silicone ice cube trays and refrigerate until almost set.
4. Once almost set, add walnut halves to the top of each fat bomb.
5. Return to fridge until firm.
6. Remove from silicone molds and store in an airtight container in the fridge for up to a week.

Servings: 14

Nutrition Facts (per serving)

Total Carbohydrates: 2,5g

Dietary Fiber:1g

Net Carbs: 1g

Protein: 0,7g

Total Fat: 10g

Calories: 88,5

Author Notes

Walnuts have been touted as one of the world's most healthiest foods. Research shows that walnut consumption may support brain health and improve cell function. They contain a good amount of healthy omega-3 fats and are delicious to boot!

Coconut and Matcha Truffles

Ingredients

For the truffles:

1 cup firm coconut oil (refrigerate if necessary)

1 cup coconut butter

1/2 cup full fat coconut milk, refrigerated overnight

1/2 tsp matcha green tea powder

1/4 tsp cinnamon

1/4 tsp sea salt

1 tsp pure vanilla extract

For the truffle coating:

1 cup finely shredded, unsweetened coconut

1 Tbs matcha green tea powder

Directions

1. Combine all of the truffle ingredients in a medium sized mixing bowl. Note that it's very important for your coconut oil be firm so send it to the fridge for a little bit if you have to. Same goes for the coconut milk - the thick cream will rise to the top and coconut water will sink to the bottom. While it's not mandatory that you use only the cream part, your milk should be very firm when you use it so make sure that you cool the can overnight.
2. Mix on high speed with a hand mixer, until light and fluffy, then place in the refrigerator to firm up for about an hour.

3. While the truffle mixture is firming up, combine the shredded coconut and matcha powder together in a large, shallow dish. Set aside.
4. With the help of a small cookie scoop form the cold truffle mixture into 32 little balls, roughly the size of a ping pong ball.
5. Roll the balls quickly between the palms of your hands to shape them into perfect little spheres, then drop each ball into the coconut/matcha mixture and roll them until completely coated.
6. Transfer your finished fat bomb balls to an airtight container and keep refrigerated for up to 2 weeks.
7. These can be eaten straight out of the fridge but taste best when you let them sit at room temperature for 10 to 15 minutes before to eat them.

Servings: 32

Nutrition Facts (per serving)

Total Carbohydrates: 0,6g

Dietary Fiber: 0,3g

Net Carbs: 0,2g

Protein: 0,2g

Total Fat: 14g

Calories: 123

Coconut-Raspberry Fat Bombs

Ingredients

1/2 cup coconut butter

1/2 cup coconut oil

1/2 cup freeze dried raspberries

1/2 cup unsweetened shredded coconut

1/4 powdered sugar substitute such as Swerve or Truvia

Directions

1. Line an 8"x8" pan with parchment paper.
2. In a food processor, coffee grinder, or blender, pulse the dried raspberries into a fine powder.
3. In a saucepan over medium heat, combine the coconut butter, coconut oil, coconut, and sweetener. Stir until melted and well combined.
4. Remove pan from heat and stir in raspberry powder.
5. Pour mixture into pan and refrigerate or freeze for several hours, or overnight.
6. Cut into 12 pieces and serve!

Servings: 12

Nutrition Facts (per serving)

Total Carbohydrates: 3,2g

Dietary Fiber: 0,8g

Net Carbs: 2,5g

Protein: 0,3g

Total Fat: 18g

Calories: 169

Author Notes

Raspberries contain antioxidants such as Vitamin C, quercetin and gallic acid which help to prevent circulatory disease and age-related decline. They are also high in ellagic acid which has been shown to have anti-inflammatory properties.

Peanut Butter Fudge

Ingredients

1 cup all natural creamy peanut butter

1 cup coconut oil

1/4 cup unsweetened vanilla almond milk

a pinch of coarse sea salt

1 tsp vanilla extract

2 tsp liquid stevia (optional)

Directions

1. In a microwave safe bowl, soften the peanut butter and coconut oil together. (About 1 minute on med-low heat.)
2. Combine the softened peanut butter and coconut oil with the remaining ingredients into a blender or food processor.
3. Blend until thoroughly combined.
4. Pour into a 9X4" loaf pan that has been lined with parchment paper.
5. Refrigerate until set. About 2 hours.
6. Enjoy!

Servings: 12

Cooking Times: 15 minutes

Nutrition Facts (per serving)

Total Carbohydrates: 4,25g

Dietary Fiber: 1,3g

Net Carbs: 2g

Protein: 5,4g

Total Fat: 29g

Calories: 284

Author Notes

Coconut oil has a multitude of health benefits including improving glucose tolerance and decreasing risk of cardiovascular disease.

Conclusion

Thank you again for purchasing this book!

I hope this Low Carb book helps you understand the Low Carb diet dynamics and principles, why you should do it and how it's going to change your outlook on food and healthy living.

The next step is to get into the right frame of mind and decide that it's time to take charge of your eating habits and your entire life in general.

Even if you have never tried the Low Carb diet before, you can do it and I can promise you one thing, after the 30 days, you will be kicking yourself for having not discovered this sooner.

I hope it was able to inspire you to clean up your diet and ditch the high-carb, low nutrient, toxic food that we, as a society, have come to accept.

The Low Carb diet is definitely a change in lifestyle that may be difficult at times, but by making these changes, you'll discover increased energy, decreased hunger, and a boosted metabolism.

I encourage you to share these recipes with family and friends, tell them about this book, and let them know that a Low Carb Diet can be delicious and nutritious.

Finally, if you feel that you have received any value from this book, then I'd like to ask if you would be kind enough to click on the link below and leave a review on Amazon to share your positive experience with other readers.
It'd be greatly appreciated!

counselling. The information presented herein has not been evaluated by the U.S Food & Drug Administration, and it is not intended to diagnose, treat, cure or prevent any disease. Full medical clearance from a licensed physician should be obtained before beginning or modifying any diet, exercise or lifestyle program, and physician should be informed of all nutritional changes. The author claims no responsibility to any person or entity for any liability, loss or damage caused or alleged to be caused directly or indirectly as a result of the use, application or interpretation of the information presented herein.

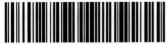

Made in the USA
Middletown, DE
06 July 2016